Mentorship in Academic Medicine

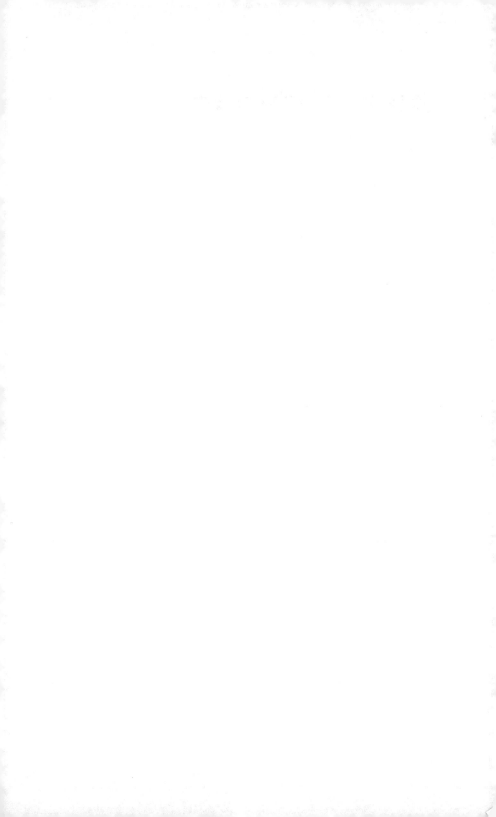

Mentorship in Academic Medicine

Sharon E. Straus MD, FRCPC, MSc

Li Ka Shing Knowledge Institute
St. Michael's Hospital;
Department of Medicine
University of Toronto
Toronto, ON
Canada

David L. Sackett OC, MD, FRSC, FRCP

Director, Trout Research & Education Centre
Irish Lake, ON
Canada

WILEY Blackwell   BMJ|Books

Library of Congress Cataloging-in-Publication Data
Straus, Sharon E., author.
  Mentorship in academic medicine / Sharon E. Straus and David L. Sackett.
    p. ; cm.
  Includes bibliographical references and index.
  ISBN 978-1-118-44602-7 (pbk.)
  I. Sackett, David L., author. II. Title.
  [DNLM: 1. Mentors. 2. Education, Medical. 3. Faculty, Medical. WB 18]
  R735.A1
  610.71 – dc23
                                                2013022741

A catalogue record for this book is available from the British Library.

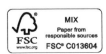

Contents

Acknowledgements

We have learned a huge amount from our mentors, mentees, friends, and colleagues about mentorship and we thank them for their ongoing support and inspiration. We thank Jennifer Deevy for obtaining permissions to reproduce some of the tables in this book, and we thank David Newton both for his hard work in organizing our mentorship survey results, and for his genius in creating the website (www.mentorshipacademicmedicine.com) that accompanies this book. Dario Sambunjak and Mitch Feldman generously provided both insights and feedback on early drafts of Chapters 6 and 7 respectively. Vic Neufeld, Donald Cole, and Lehana Thabane reviewed drafts of the book and provided us with thoughtful feedback on its contents.

We thank each of our amazing colleagues who not only serve as role models of excellent mentorship, but took the time to tell us how they did it through completion of a survey (and are allowing us to share their insights and expertise with you). They include: Paul Armstrong, Jesse Berlin, Mohit Bhandari, Dianne Bryant, John Cairns, Bill Clark, Rebecca Clarke, Deborah Cook, Gary Cutter, Dave Davis, Simon Day, Julian Desmond, John Eikelboom, Justin Ezekowitz, Brian Feldman, Amit Garg, Hertzel Gerstein, Paul Glasziou, Christian Gluud, Charles Goldsmith, Vladimir Hachinski, Robert Hart, Brian Haynes, Brenda Hemmelgarn, Carl Heneghan, Asbjørn Hróbjartsson, Clive Kearon, Andreas Laupacis, France Légaré, Sandy MacPherson, Bonani Mayosi, Maureen Meade, Cindy Mulrow, Jock Murray, Jim Neaton, Andy Oxman, Barry Pless, Don Redelmeier, Roberta Scherer, David Simel, Peter Szatmari, Shaun Treweek, Andrew Vickers, Allyn Walsh, and James Ware.

Sharon would like to particularly thank her family for their patience and support. She gives special thanks to Jeremy Grimshaw, Brian Haynes, Andreas Laupacis, and Arthur Slutsky who continue to provide her with mentorship.

Much of Dave's contribution to this book is an expansion of his 'Clinician-trialist rounds' column in the journal *Clinical Trials*, and he thanks its editor, Steve Goodman, for shepherding that enterprise. Individual "rounds" were guest-led by Sharon, Peter Szatmari, and Andy Oxman, and frequently incorporated comments from fellow trialists the world 'round.

Introduction

We reckon that few academics would argue against the importance of mentorship in academic medicine; after all, you're reading this introduction! As we hope to convince you in Chapter 1, effective mentorship is a major determinant of academic success and both job and life satisfaction. However, although most studies of academic faculty suggest that they want mentorship [1–3], there are lots of academic settings in which less than 20% of them get it. In recognition of this yawning gap, many academic health institutions are developing mentorship programs and, in doing so, have recognized the paucity of educational as well as administrative resources to educate and support both mentors and mentees. We wrote this book to help meet this need.

How did we get interested in mentorship?

Sharon became interested in mentorship while completing a research fellowship at the University of Oxford under Dave's supervision. At their first meeting, Dave asked her to outline her career goals as well as those for her research training. Dave's response changed her life: he told her that his job was to make sure she achieved what she wanted in her fellowship and to support her in the development of her career path. This altruism was role modeled throughout the next few years and Dave's amazing mentorship skills and expertise directly influenced her career and her own attempts at mentorship. When preparing to leave Oxford and begin her first faculty position, Sharon asked Dave how she could ever repay him for what he'd given to her and his immediate response was, "Do the same for others." Now, after mentoring more than 50 graduate students and new faculty, Sharon states that one of the most fulfilling parts of her job is to be able to interact with and learn from her mentees. It is these experiences, plus the scarcity of resources describing how to develop and support mentorship, that led to several research projects and, ultimately, to this book.

Dave, akin to Molière's Monsieur Jourdain*, was getting mentored for years before he knew it. Beginning in a US medical school in 1958 (back when man still had 48 chromosomes), and in his internship, first medical residency, and nephrology fellowship, he was "adopted" in turn by a bench scientist, a chair of medicine, and a nephrologist who didn't simply recruit him into their bailiwicks as an extra brain and pair of hands to be "supervised." Instead, and in turn, they took time each week or so to challenge his ways of thinking about what he "knew" and might be able to find out about human biology and clinical medicine, to open doors to the places ("restricted" labs and graduate courses) where he might learn how to find those things out, to critique and improve his plebeian writing and speaking skills, to explore his career interests and ambitions, and to help him think how he might pursue them through his next career moves. Twenty-five years later, after getting educated about mentoring and instituting it at a new Canadian medical and graduate school, his seventh mentor helped him think through and implement his second medicine residency. He's now on his tenth mentor and gazillionth mentee, and beginning to get the hang of it [4].

Who are the potential readers of this book?

We have written this book for aspiring academic researchers and educators (whom we'll hereafter call *mentees*) and those experienced, empathic persons who guide them in the development and re-examination of their own ideas, learning, and personal and professional development (whom we'll call *mentors*). We are academic physicians (namely, we are subspecialists in internal medicine and geriatric medicine and don't presume to be experts in other clinical areas) who have largely worked in North America and the UK. Most of our mentees have been physicians, but we have mentored people from various disciplines including nursing, medicine, rehabilitation therapy, biostatistics, health informatics, education, and engineering amongst others and from different career paths including clinician educators, researchers, and administrators. While there is some material in this book that is relevant to anyone working in an academic institution, we don't to pretend to be experts in mentorship for other types of clinicians and academics (such as those in other clinical disciplines or career paths) or for those working in low and middle income countries, and we encourage them to identify (or create) mentorship resources that outline issues unique to their mentorship needs. We invite these readers to share these resources

---

* . . . who exclaimed: "Well, what do you know about that! These forty years now I've been speaking in prose without knowing it!" Molière: *The Bourgeois Gentleman*, 1670.

with us via our website (www.mentorshipacademicmedicine.com) and to lead discussions on the website about which contents from the book are useful to them and which ones aren't relevant. In the literature review that we conducted to inform this book, most of the articles focused on mentorship for clinician scientists. We found less research that targeted clinician educators and clinician administrators and thus our discussion of mentorship for academics following these career paths is not exhaustive. Again, we encourage our readers to send any relevant research targeting these individuals to our website.

We have targeted our book primarily at mentoring in academic institutions. Accordingly, we have viewed our readers and their interests, goals, aspirations, opportunities, resources, challenges, and dilemmas through that lens, and at both the individual and institutional levels:

- At the individual mentor–mentee level, we've presented the best evidence we could find on what they should look for in each other, how they should find each other, how they should treat each other, how they should plan and run their mentoring sessions, and how they should identify and manage the opportunities, challenges, and problems mentees encounter as they launch their academic careers (including how to fix or sever mentorships that aren't working).
- At the institutional level, we've presented the best evidence we could find on how to assess an institution's need for and interest in mentoring, how to develop a mentoring program and train mentors, and how to evaluate it, correct its faults, and sustain it. While most of the literature focuses on clinician scientists, we have included information for other career paths whenever we have found it. Similarly, although most of the evidence focuses on mentoring trainees and junior faculty, we've addressed issues for senior faculty whenever possible.

Is this book about the theory or practice of mentorship?

There are some brilliant people who are continuing to develop a theoretical basis for mentoring [5, 6]: we are not among them. This book is about the practice of mentoring.

How is this book organised?

This book employs a case-stimulus learning approach:
- Each chapter begins with a scenario for the reader to ponder and solve.
- Next, comes the best evidence we could find about the issues raised in the scenario.

- Finally, we close with some evidence-based, actionable solutions to the challenges presented in the scenario.

Where did we get the evidence for the material in this book?

We identified the evidence in each chapter from three sources:

1 Our systematic reviews and updates of the mentorship literature. Updates since this book went to press can be found on our website.

2 Our 2012 survey of international colleagues who have been recognized by their peers as being excellent mentors. We identified 271 colleagues from various academic settings around the world who have been active in various career pathways and have some expertise as a mentor. We invited them to complete a survey, either electronically or via phone interview, and to share their thoughts on targets for effective mentorship, tips for achieving these targets, potential mentorship problems, and strategies for overcoming these problems. Forty-five colleagues responded to our request and we have incorporated their anonymized responses in this book. We have posted the survey on our website that accompanies this book (www.mentorshipacademicmedicine.com) and we invite readers to take a few minutes to review it and share their answers to the survey with us.

3 Our own experiences as mentors, mentees and developers of institution-level mentorship programs.

Because the GRADE system [7] doesn't yet have a scale for assessing qualitative literature, we used a modified version to describe the validity and "trustability" of the evidence we present in each chapter. In brief, we labelled evidence as *high quality* when we are highly confident that the true effect of the mentoring intervention lies close to that estimated in the publication. For example, evidence is judged as high quality if all of the following apply:

- there is a wide range of studies included in the analyses with no major limitations
- there is little variation between studies
- the summary estimate has a narrow confidence interval.

We judge evidence as *moderate quality* when we consider the true effect is likely to be close to the published estimate of the effect, but there is a possibility that it is substantially different. For example, evidence might be judged as moderate quality if any of the following applies:

- there are only a few studies and some have limitations but not major flaws
- there is some variation between studies
- the confidence interval of the summary estimate is wide.

Finally, we judge evidence to be *low quality* when the true effect may be substantially different from the published estimate of its effect. For example, evidence might be judged as low quality if any of the following apply:
- the studies have major methodological flaws
- there is important variation between study results
- the confidence interval of the summary estimate of the effect is very wide [7, 8].

What other mentorship resources are available to complement this book?

We are supplementing and updating the contents of this book on our website at www.mentorshipacademicmedicine.com. As this book was being published, it included:
- a mentorship checklist
- an individual development plan
- interviews with various mentors
- some mentorship scenarios.

A major portion of this website will provide updates of new evidence for each chapter so that readers can see what's new or different since the book was published. We'll update this evidence-base by repeating our systematic reviews. Furthermore, we'll translate any new, valid evidence into new, effective strategies and tactics for mentees, mentors, and institutions.

We invite you, our readers, to take over[†] the website.
- When you come across moderate- or high-quality evidence on mentoring that we missed in preparing this book, please add it to the website. For example, we've worked mostly in academic centers in high-income countries, and we'd welcome contributions from colleagues who are mentoring in other settings such as those in low-income countries.
- When you have had a particularly positive or negative experience in mentoring or being mentored, please add it to the respective chapter, telling the rest of us what you think its "active" principle was so that we can duplicate or discard it accordingly.
- When you find important gaps that we simply failed to cover, let us know.
- And we always appreciate having this book's errors (including typos, misspellings, and other goofs) identified and corrected.

[†] The usual standards for website participation will be employed, and you are free to sign your contributions (and be acknowledged for them) or remain anonymous.

References

1. Genuardi FJ, Zenni EA. Adolescent medicine faculty development needs. J Adolesc Health 2001; 29: 46–49.
2. Wise MR, Shapiro H, Bodley J, *et al.* Factors affecting academic promotion in obstetrics and gynaecology in Canada. J Obstet Gynaecol Can 2004; 26: 127–136.
3. Palepu A, Friedman RH, Barnett RC, *et al.* Junior faculty members' mentoring relationships and their professional development in U.S. medical schools. Acad Med 1998; 73: 318–323.
4. Sackett DL. On the determinants of academic success as a clinician-scientist. Clin Invest Med 2001; 24: 94–100.
5. Ragins BR, Kram KE. *The Handbook of Mentoring at Work: Theory, Research and Practice.* Thousand Oaks, CA: Sage Publications, 2007.
6. Bozeman B, Feeney MK. Towards a useful theory of mentoring. Adm Soc 2007; 39: 719–30.
7. Guyatt GH, Oxman AD, Vist GE, *et al.* GRADE: An emerging consensus on rating quality of evidence and strength of recommendations. BMJ 2008; 336: 924–6.
8. GRADE Working Group. Available from: http://www.gradeworkinggroup.org/ Accessed Sept 20, 2012.

Chapter 1 What is the evidence for mentorship?

Scenario

At the end of your first year as an academic clinician–investigator in a big, busy clinical department, with some 200 faculty members, you've just finished discussing your annual review with your department chair. She tells you that you're doing extremely well for a new faculty member, which is a great relief to you. Although you think you've done pretty well – in the past year, you received a peer-reviewed development grant, first-authored two papers and co-authored four others, have a systematic review in press, have an abstract accepted for a national meeting, are enjoying your time on the clinical service, and the medical students and residents submitted glowing assessments of your bedside teaching – you feel pressed for time, worry about your work–life balance, and wonder whether you're "on the right track" for a successful and enjoyable academic career. Although you've received encouragement from several senior members of the department, you've been conscious of how busy they are and don't want to impose on their jam-packed schedules to ask for advice. But now, stimulated by a recent session on mentoring which you attended at an academic meeting and emboldened by your chair's praise, you tell her that you and some of your colleagues are concerned about the lack of a formal mentorship program in the department. She says that to be able to "sell" this idea to the department, she wants to see the evidence that such a program does more than waste time, money, and energy, and she challenges you to lead a working group to track down, appraise, and summarize the evidence that a formal mentoring program benefits the career development and life-satisfaction of academic clinicians. With the promise of some staff support for your working group, you accept her challenge.

Your first step in this task is to gather the evidence; specifically, what's the case for mentorship?

In this chapter, we'll set the stage for our mentorship discussion providing the definitions and terminology that we'll use throughout this book. In particular,

Mentorship in Academic Medicine, First Edition. Sharon E. Straus and David L. Sackett.
© 2014 John Wiley & Sons, Ltd. Published 2014 by John Wiley & Sons, Ltd.

we'll outline the scope for our discussion, including what mentorship is and isn't, and help you to provide the "case for mentorship" based on the relevant evidence. We invite you to join us in this dialogue via the website (www.mentorshipacademicmedicine.com) that accompanies this book; we'd love to hear about how you define mentorship and how you would meet the challenge we posed in the above scenario!*

What is mentorship?

The concept of mentorship can be traced to Greek methodology. Odysseus placed his much older friend Mentor in charge of his palace and of his son Telemachus when he left for the Trojan War. Interestingly, Athena disguised herself as Mentor on several occasions to provide guidance to Telemachus. It was from this story that the term "mentor" was taken and began being used to mean a trusted, senior advisor who provides guidance to a more junior person.

Moving along to more recent times, there are many definitions of mentorship, including those from business [1] and psychology literature [2], but our focus in this book is on academic medicine, including clinicians who work in universities and academic health science centres. So, for our discussion, we'll use the definition commonly cited in academic medical literature:

> A process whereby an experienced, highly regarded, empathetic person (the mentor) guides another (usually younger or more junior) individual (the mentee[†]) in the development and re-examination of their own ideas, learning, and personal and professional development. The mentor, who often (but not necessarily) works in the same organization or field as the mentee, achieves this by listening or talking in confidence to the mentee [3].

One element that we think is missing from this definition is that mentorship is about an exchange between the mentor and mentee and provides benefits to both parties; we'll explore these benefits later in this chapter.

Berk and colleagues have further elucidated the concept of mentorship to specify that it can range from an informal, short-term relationship to a formal, long-term relationship [4]. *Informal* mentoring is a relationship between individuals that develops without organizational interventions and

---

* There are different ways of tackling this challenge and we've provided our proposed solution to this scenario at the end of this chapter.
† Note that we use the term "mentee" to refer to the target of mentorship. In the literature, protégé is a term that is sometimes used interchangeably, but we find this term paternalistic and will stick to mentee in this book.

is the natural "coming together" of a mentor and mentee. For example, a resident may identify a staff physician with whom they worked on a clinical rotation and developed a good rapport; this interaction may lead to a series of conversations that ultimately results in a mentoring relationship. *Formal* mentoring is initiated (in some places, mandated!) by an outside party or organization, as when a department chair not only requires that each new recruit has a mentor but makes sure that they get one.

A common source of confusion in the mentorship literature is that the term "mentor" is often used interchangeably with the term "role model" or "coach." We maintain that these are very different concepts. "Role modeling" is a "passive, observational learning model in which an individual attempts to emulate observed, desirable behaviours and qualities" [5]. Indeed, there may be no personal relationship with the role model, and they are often oblivious of their role! Of course, a mentor can and often does serve as a role model, but that's just one, passive facet of their function. Similarly, mentoring goes far beyond "coaching" a junior colleague on the performance of specific tasks and skills [6]. This latter function is often the complete extent of an aspiring academic clinician's interactions with their research supervisor or department chair. We found an interesting analogy (for anyone who has seen Star Wars) that nicely highlights this difference: "Yoda is a coach, teaching Luke how to use the Force, and Obi-Wan Kenobi is a mentor, showing him what it means to be a Jedi knight" [7].

Who are the targets for mentorship?

Much of the literature on mentorship focuses on targeting junior or new faculty members [8–10]. However, faculty at any stage in their career can benefit from it.[‡] A large qualitative study (moderate-quality evidence) of clinician researchers across two universities documented that senior (or established) faculty often feel that they are neglected and should have equitable access to mentors [11]. We also found a descriptive study of a mentorship program developed in a Department of Pediatrics at an academic medical centre that targeted mentorship activities not only to junior, but to mid-career and senior faculty [12]. Their survey of mid-career (associate professor level) department members found that respondents commonly wanted mentoring around the requirements and timelines for promotion, about how to redefine their careers, and how to network effectively (they were less interested in advice from mentors on how to transition to

---

[‡] Dave Sackett linked up with his first mentor in 1958 and is currently mentee to his tenth.

administrative positions) [12]. Senior faculty wanted mentoring around how to transition towards part-time opportunities and retirement, and on financial and succession planning. These results highlight that as a mentee's career progresses and evolves to take on different responsibilities or change career paths, different sorts of mentoring may be required. For example, a mentee's emerging interest in administration or education may require mentoring skills beyond those of their earlier clinician–scientist mentor.

In academic medicine, clinicians can have different career paths including those of a scientist, educator, or administrator, and having this career flexibility is one of the privileges and pleasures of academic medicine. Interestingly, surveys and qualitative literature (moderate-quality evidence) suggest that clinician investigators are both more likely to seek mentorship and more comfortable asking for it than are clinician educators [8–10]. This difference may be because clinician investigators have completed research training, are already used to having research supervisors, and are "primed" to seek the greater benefits of mentors. These studies also suggest that clinician educators are more likely to have difficulty with promotion than clinician scientists, raising the possibility of a causal relationship [8–10]. Throughout this book, we will identify differences in mentorship issues for each of these career paths whenever we find them in the literature.

What is the impact of mentorship?

Mentorship claims to develop and maintain faculty who are productive, satisfied, collegial, and socially responsible. However, not only are there no randomized trials of mentorship; we doubt we will ever see one, since it would be both methodologically and ethically challenging to randomize clinicians to either receive a mentor or be denied access to one.[§] Accordingly, we based this section on the results from three systematic reviews of the literature [8–10], updated by more recent literature searches to the first week of March 2012. Studies of any design were eligible for inclusion, but the final selection was restricted to English-language reports targeting academic medical faculty.

Much of the evidence base is summarized in a quantitative systematic review that explored the impact of mentoring on career choices and academic advancement [8]. It included 42 articles describing 39 studies (34 of which were cross-sectional self-report surveys). A second systematic review of the

---

[§] On the other hand, if we can identify enough academic centers with an interest in mentorship but no programs, a stepped wedge cluster randomized trial could provide powerful evidence on whether it works. We'd be keen to hear from any programs that might be interested in tackling this challenge!

qualitative literature on mentorship identified 9 relevant studies [9]. Since the publication of these reviews, we identified an additional 13 eligible studies:
- 7 surveys [13–19]
- 2 nested case control studies [20, 21]
- 1 uncontrolled before-and-after study [22]
- 1 case series [23]
- 2 qualitative studies [24, 25].

Most of the evidence base comes from cross-sectional surveys of academic clinicians who had or had not been previously mentored. The methodological shortcomings of such studies must be recognized. Specifically, if mentored academics are more successful in these observational studies, possible explanations for their success extend beyond mentoring, and include the possibility that they were destined to be stars from birth and therefore had a selection advantage in getting access to superior training programs that provided coincidental but unnecessary mentoring. And, the majority of the studies that we've found to date were done at a single site and didn't follow mentees' careers over a sufficiently long period of time.

Bearing these caveats in mind, there appear to be career- and life-benefits of mentorship to both mentors and mentees. We'll explore the benefits to mentees first:

1 *Academic clinicians who got mentored reported greater career satisfaction* [moderate quality evidence; 14–16, 22, 26]. Mentorship not only influences career choice [10, 24], it influences job satisfaction. For example, in a survey of faculty from 24 US medical schools, faculty members with mentors had significantly higher career-satisfaction scores (62.6 vs 59.5 on a 100-point scale, $p < 0.003$) than those without mentors [26]. Similarly, in a survey of gastroenterologists in the US, having a mentor was a predictor of job satisfaction (odds ratio of 2.32, $p < 0.001$) [15]. And, in a survey of mentors and mentees from the Psychiatry Institute at King's College, London, having a mentor was associated with greater job well-being [22]. In contrast, Stamm and Buddeberg-Fischer have followed a cohort of Swiss medical school graduates for more than seven years with both repeated surveys and a nested case-control study and showed that having a mentor was not predictive of job satisfaction [20]. However, mentorship did predict self-perceived career success [20].

2 *Academic clinicians who were mentored got more research grants* [moderate quality evidence; 27, 28]. Mentorship can enhance productivity. For example, a survey within a nested case-control study found that mentored primary care fellows were two to three times as likely to be a principal investigator on a research grant [28].

3 *Academic clinicians who were mentored reported more protected time for scholarly activities and produced more publications* [moderate quality evidence; 17, 26, 29–31]. A survey of more than 3000 faculty members in the US found that those with a mentor had more time allocated to research (28% vs 15%, $p < 0.001$) than those who didn't have a mentor [26]. In another study, survey respondents who had a mentor were more likely to allocate more time to research and were more productive in research in terms of their numbers of grants and publications [28].

4 *Academic clinicians who were mentored were promoted more quickly* [moderate quality evidence; 8, 18, 32]. Not surprisingly, given that mentorship is associated with greater productivity of academic outputs, mentorship seems to facilitate academic promotion. For example, a study of Canadian obstetrics and gynecology fellows found that those who reported that they had a mentor were more likely to achieve a promotion (hazard ratio 2.3; 95% confidence interval 1.36–3.99) [32]. Surveys in the US, Canada, and Germany found that the absence of effective mentoring was a major obstacle to a successful academic career [8]. In a small survey of 12 faculty, Daley and colleagues found that having a senior mentor was a factor in determining promotion [18].

5 *Academics who were mentored were more likely to stay at their academic institutions* [moderate quality evidence; 33]. Mentorship may play a key role in recruiting and retaining staff in academic medicine. For example, in a two-tiered program consisting of one year of preceptoring new faculty (to orient them) plus mentoring junior faculty who had been there for at least a year, 38% of junior faculty who did not form mentor partnerships left the organization, compared with 15% of those who did [33].

6 *Academic clinicians who were mentored reported greater academic "self-efficacy"* [moderate quality evidence; 13, 22]. Academic self-efficacy is defined as the belief in one's ability to succeed in academic medicine. A survey of faculty members at the University of California, San Francisco reported that those who had a mentor reported significantly greater academic self-efficacy than those without mentors [13]. Similarly, Dutta and colleagues found that having a mentor was associated with both self-efficacy and self-esteem [22].

There is less literature available on the impact of mentorship on mentors, and we identified just two recent studies that explored this issue [22, 34]. In a survey of mentors for medical students, mentorship was reported to reinvigorate interest and lead to personal and professional growth [34]. In their before-and-after study, Dutta and colleagues documented mentors' enjoyment in being able to help solve mentees' problems, "to give back," provide support, see their mentees develop, and in using the mentorship to reflect on their own careers and skills [22].

Gaps in the evidence

As we emphasized at the outset, there are no randomized trials of mentoring. While completing a multi-centered randomized trial of mentorship would be challenging, we repeat our invitation to colleagues who might wish to collaborate in designing and executing the stepped wedge cluster randomized trial described earlier in this chapter. Short of this, longer-term cohort studies of aspiring academics, with and without mentors, which examine the impact of mentorship on the retention, productivity, ability to mentor others, quality of life, and satisfaction of mentees would shed important additional light on its risks and benefits.

Bottom line and scenario resolution

We conclude that effective mentorship is vital to career success. It produces benefits for both mentors and mentees. Conversely, we conclude that absent or failed mentorship leads to lower productivity and hampers the ability to achieve career benchmarks and personal growth. In the next few chapters of this book, we will present some ways to think about mentors, mentees, mentoring strategies and tactics, and how to develop and monitor a mentorship program.

Returning to the scenario that opened this chapter:

1 You develop a working group of 8 to 10 colleagues from your department including those from different career paths (clinician educators, investigators, administrators) and rank (assistant, associate, and full professor). You use purposive sampling to ensure that you include colleagues who are perceived as being opinion leaders in your faculty and who could be champions for this initiative, and include skeptics as well as proponents of mentorship.

2 After circulating, discussing, and debating the evidence, your working group concludes that mentoring does far more good than harm to both mentees and mentors, and ought to be systematically implemented in your department. You create a one-page summary with key messages that outline your conclusions. If accepted by your chair, these messages will form the rationale for your mentorship strategy and will be used to engage others in the mentorship program.

3 You present your report to your chair, who – after vigorous debate – is won over by both the quality of your review and the strength of your conclusions.

4 She agrees to support you in carrying out a "needs assessment" with your faculty members to begin to better understand the need for mentorship amongst your colleagues. As a result, your working group conducts a survey

to determine how many faculty members currently have a mentor, want a mentor, are a mentor, or are interested in becoming a mentor.

5 Your survey documents widespread dissatisfaction with the current, informal "hit-and-miss" mentoring that exists in the department, and widespread advocacy of an organized mentoring program with the initial goal of providing mentors to every senior trainee and all new faculty.

6 Your chair agrees to fund a start-up mentoring program (including support staff).

7 Finally, your chair sends formal letters of commendation to you and your committee members for you to add to your promotion and tenure dossier.

References

1. Kram KE. Mentoring at work: developmental relationships in organizational life. Glenview: Scott Foresman, 1985.

2. Levinson DJ, Darrow CN, Klein EB, *et al. The Seasons of a Man's Life.* New York: Knopf, 1978.

3. Standing Committee on Postgraduate Medical and Dental Education. Supporting doctors and dentists at work: an enquiry into mentoring. 1998. Available from: www.mcgl.dircon.co.uk/scopme/mentor5.pdf. Accessed 24 April 2012.

4. Berk RA, Berg J, Mortimer R, *et al.* Measuring the effectiveness of faculty mentoring relationships. Acad Med 2005; 80: 66–71.

5. Donovan A. Views of radiology program directors on the role of mentorship in the training of radiology resident. AJR 2010; 194: 704–8.

6. Fielden SL, Davidson M, Sutherland VJ. Innovations in coaching and mentoring. Health Services Man Res 2009; 22: 92–9.

7. Management Mentors. An example of a good mentor. Available from: http://www.management-mentors.com/about/corporate-mentoring-matters-blog/bid/17517/An-example-of-a-good-mentor. Accessed 24 April 2012.

8. Sambunjak D, Straus SE, Marusic A. Mentoring in academic medicine: a systematic review. JAMA 2006; 296; 1103–15.

9. Sambunjak D, Straus SE, Marusic A. A systematic review of qualitative research of the meaning and characteristics of mentoring in academic medicine. J Gen Int Med 2010; 25: 72–8.

10. Straus SE, Straus C, Tzanetos K. Career choice in academic medicine: a systematic review. J Gen Int Med 2006; 21: 1222–9.

11. Straus SE, Chatur F, Taylor M. Issues in the mentor-mentee relationship in academic medicine: qualitative study. Acad Med 2009; 84: 135–9.

12. Schor NK, Guillet R, McAnarney ER. Anticipatory guidance as a principle of faculty development: managing transition and change. Acad Med 2011; 86: 1235–40.

13. Feldman MD, Huang L, Guglielmo BJ, *et al.* Training the next generation of research mentors. Clin Trans Sci 2009; 2: 216-21.

14. Chung KC, Song JW, Kim HM, *et al.* Predictors of job satisfaction among academic faculty members: Do institutional and clinical staff differ? Med Ed 2010; 44: 985–95.

15. Travis AC, Katz PO, Kane SV. Mentoring in gastroenterology. Am J Gasteroenterol 2010; 105; 970–2.

16. Wasserstein AG, Quistberg A, Shea JA. Mentoring at the University of Pennsylvania: Results of a faculty survey. J Gen Int Med 2007; 22: 210–4.

17. Kaderli R, Muff B, Stefenelli U, Businger A. Female surgeons' mentoring experiences and success in an academic career in Switzerland. Swiss Med Wkly 2011; 18: 141.

18. Daley SP, Broyles SL, Rivera LM, *et al.* A conceptual model for faculty development in academic medicine: The underrepresented minority faculty experience. J Natl Med Assoc 2011; 103: 816–21.

19. Anderson MS, Horn AS, Risbey KR, *et al.* What do mentoring and training in the responsible conduct of research have to do with scientists' behavior. Acad Med 2007; 82: 853–6.

20. Stamm M, Buddeberg-Fischer B. The impact of mentoring during postgraduate training on doctors' career success. Med Educ 2011; 45: 488–96

21. Orandi BJ, Blackburn S, Henke PK. Surgical mentors' and mentees' productivity from 1993 to 2006. Am J Surg 2011; 201: 260–3.

22. Dutta R, Hawkes SL, Kuipers E, *et al.* One year outcomes of a mentoring scheme for female academics: a pilot study at the Institute of Psychiatry, King's College London. BMC Med Educ 2011; 11: 13.

23. Interian A, Escobar J. The use of a mentoring-based conference as a research career stimulation strategy. Acad Med 2009; 84: 1389–94.

24. Borges NJ, Navarro AM, Grover AC. Women physicians: choosing a career in academic medicine. Acad Med 2012; 87: 105–14.

25. Taylor CA, Taylor JC, Stoller JK. The influence of mentorship and role modeling on developing physician-leaders: views of aspiring and established physician-leaders. J Gen Intern Med 2009; 24: 1130–4.

26. Palepu A, Friedman RH, Barnett RC, *et al.* Junior faculty members' mentoring relationships and their professional development in U.S. medical schools. Acad Med 1998; 73: 318–23.

27. Curtis P, Dickinson P, Steiner J, *et al.* Building capacity for research in family medicine: is the blueprint faulty? Fam Med 2003; 35: 124–30.

28. Steiner JF, Curtis P, Lanphear B, Vu KO. Assessing the role of influential mentors in the research development of primary care fellows. Acad Med 2004; 79: 865–72.

29. Illes J, Glover GH, Wexler L, *et al.* A model for faculty mentoring in academic radiology. Acad Radiol 2007; 7: 717–24.

30. Levinson W, Kaufman K, Clark B, Tolle S. Mentors and role models for women in academic medicine. West J Med 1991; 154: 423–6.

31. Pearlman S, Leef K, Sciscione AC. Factors that affect satisfaction with neonatal-perinatal fellowship training. Am J Perinatol 2004; 21: 371–5.

32. Wise MR, Shapiro H, Bodley J, *et al.* Factors affecting academic promotion in obstetrics and gynecology in Canada. J Obstetr Gynecol Can 2004; 26: 127–36.

33. Benson CA, Morahan PS, Sachdeva AK, Richman RC. Effective faculty precep-
    toring and mentoring during reorganization of an academic medical center. Med
    Teach 2002; 24: 550–57.
34. Stenfors-Hayes, Kalen S, Hult H, *et al.* Being a mentor for undergraduate medical
    students enhance personal and professional development. Med Teacher 2010;
    32: 148–53.

Chapter 2 What are the characteristics and behaviors of effective mentors and mentees?

Scenarios

Pick the one that best fits your current situation:

1 *For new junior faculty*: Having just completed both your clinical and advanced research/education training, you have started your first academic job. Your department chair has asked you whether you'd be willing to be a mentor to departmental graduate students. Stop reading at this point and make two lists:
   a) In terms of characteristics and behaviors, what do you think an ideal mentor should be like?
   b) If you're going to take this on, what characteristics and behaviors would you want your mentees to have?

2 *For mid-career faculty*: You are a successful mid-career researcher/educator, and your departmental chair has asked you whether you'd be willing to be a mentor to graduate students and/or new faculty members. Stop reading at this point and make two lists:
   a) In terms of characteristics and behaviors, what do you think an ideal mentor should be like?
   b) If you're going to take this on, what characteristics and behaviors would you want your mentees to have?

3 *For new graduate students*: Having completed your clinical training, today is your first day as a graduate student in applied health research/education. The program facilitates access to a mentor, and you will meet yours in a few days. Stop reading at this point and make two lists:
   a) In terms of characteristics and behaviors, what would an ideal mentor for you be like?
   b) If you're to make the most out of this mentoring opportunity, what should your behavior be like?

4 *An alternative scenario for new junior faculty*: Having completed both your clinical and advanced research/education training, today is your first day

Mentorship in Academic Medicine, First Edition. Sharon E. Straus and David L. Sackett.
© 2014 John Wiley & Sons, Ltd. Published 2014 by John Wiley & Sons, Ltd.

as a junior faculty member. The department facilitates access to a mentor, and you will meet yours in a few days. Stop reading at this point and make two lists:

a) In terms of characteristics and behaviors, what would an ideal mentor for you be like?

b) If you're to make the most out of this mentoring opportunity, what should your behavior be like?

5 *For late-career faculty*: You've had a highly successful academic career, and wonder whether seeking any (more) mentoring at your stage would be worth the time and effort. Stop reading at this point and make two lists:

a) In terms of characteristics and behaviors, what would an ideal mentor for you be like?

b) If you're to make the most out of this mentoring opportunity, what should your behavior be like?

Highly successful academics frequently credit one or a just a few of their senior colleagues for stimulating, nurturing, and greatly accelerating their professional and personal growth and development. This chapter will summarize our current understanding of those attributes and behaviors of both mentors and mentees that are most closely associated with this academic success, and how they are expressed.

As pointed out in Chapter 1, this understanding is derived from circumstantial (moderate-quality) evidence: retrospective observations from and about successful and unsuccessful academics, cross-sectional surveys of the desires and preferences of mentees, and horror-stories of mentors' theft from and abuse of their mentees.

Effective mentors

What are the characteristics of effective mentors? A recent systematic review [1] of qualitative studies among both mentors and mentees identified several qualities of effective mentors. We have updated the search since this review was published and identified and included an additional report of the qualities that led to Lifetime Achievement in Mentorship awards at the University of California, San Francisco [2]. Summarized in Table 2.1, qualities of effective mentors are of three sorts: personal attributes, behaviors toward mentees, and professional stature.

Personal attributes of effective mentors

The personal attributes of effective mentors are those that not only allow, but enable and encourage the creation of a safe environment for the frank and

Table 2.1   Characteristics of effective mentors

Dimension	Characteristic
Personal attributes	Altruistic/generous
	Enthusiastic
	Understanding/compassionate
	Nonjudgmental
	Patient
	Honest
	Responsive
	Trustworthy
	Reliable
	Excels at active listening
	Motivating
	Self-appraising
Behaviors toward mentees	Accessible
	Works hard to develop an important relationship with the mentee
	Consistently offers help in the mentee's best interests
	Identifies the mentee's potential strengths
	Assists mentees in defining and reaching their goals
	Holds a high standard for the mentee's achievements
	Compatible with mentee's practice style, vision, and personality
Professional stature	Already successful and well-respected in their field
	Well-connected to sources of additional help

Adapted from: [1] Sambunjak D, Straus SE, Marusic A. A systematic review of qualitative research on the meaning and characteristics of mentoring in academic medicine. Gen Intern Med 2010; 25: 72–8, with kind permission from Springer Science and Business Media; and [2] Cho CS, Ramanan RA, Feldman MD. Defining the ideal qualities of mentorship: A qualitative analysis of the characteristics of outstanding mentors. Am J Med 2011; 124: 453–8, with permission from Elsevier, Copyright © 2011, Elsevier.

confidential identification and exploration of all the positive and negative attitudes, hopes, fears, and experiences of mentees as they embark on academic careers.

- *Altruistic/generous*: Mentors must really like to mentor, and must be willing to devote the substantial (at times enormous) time and energy required to serve their mentees in a selfless fashion. As one former grateful mentee wrote:

> She makes little distinction between projects on which she is or is not a co-author, or between fellows or faculty with whom she has a close or distant mentoring relationship for research. For example, she has without hesitation provided me many hours of thoughtful advice on my papers and grants from which she will receive no professional recognition or benefit [2].

This altruistic, generous behavior also generates rewards for mentors. As mentioned in Chapter 1, there isn't a lot of evidence on the impact on mentors and it is largely qualitative. This evidence and our own experience suggests that mentoring can repay the past debt owed to their own mentors, can provide the thrill and pride of seeing a mentee succeed, offers the enjoyment and excitement of taking partial credit for that mentee's success, can enhance the mentor's academic reputation through spotting and developing highly talented young people, and frequently develops a dependable, collaborative junior colleague [3].

- *Enthusiastic*: Effective mentors display intense, eager, and infectious enjoyment and interest in academic health care, in the pursuit and application of new knowledge that will improve it, and in life in general. One of the most important factors for mentees choosing a career in academic medicine was exposure to an enthusiastic mentor who showed passion for their job [4].

- *Understanding/compassionate*: Effective mentors understand "where their mentee is coming from," and are deeply aware of how differences in ethnicity, language, gender, and generation can create barriers to effective mentoring [5].

- *Non-judgmental*: Effective mentors avoid forcing their own ideas about "what is best" for the career paths and development of their mentees and are non-judgemental about their mentees' values, attitudes, and aspirations. Rather, they help mentees sort these out for themselves.

- *Patient*: Mentees have different learning and working styles and effective mentors are able to diagnose these and be patient with their mentee's false-starts, rethinks, and limitations.

- *Honest*: Effective mentors are truthful in offering opinions and historic examples on the merits and likely successes (and failures) of their mentees' research ideas, protocols, papers and presentations. Always supportive, and stating major negative criticisms constructively (i.e. with suggestions for improvement), in private, away from mentees' peers and superiors, effective mentors avoid glossing over errors or ignoring their mentee's unresearchable ideas, unfundable protocols, incomprehensible manuscripts, and inscrutable presentations.

- *Responsive*: Effective mentors not only encourage their mentees to raise anything for discussion (from how to handle a political issue within their clinical department to how to arrange their schedule to make sure they can pick up their children from school), but also are able to respond to them. Because effective mentoring has to serve the entire gamut of factors affecting a mentee's career development, issues may arise that call for information or expertise beyond the knowledge or competency of their mentor. An example of the former might be the special challenges associated with parental leave brought to a childless mentor; of the latter, it might be conflicts with the on-call and on-service scheduling of a clinical department brought to a non-clinical mentor. A universal challenge for mentees is their work–life balance [6], especially in the early years when many of them are starting families, or later on when balancing the needs of aging parents. When these issues arise and are beyond their expertise, effective mentors quickly recruit knowledgeable colleagues for their expert inputs and ensure that there is transparent communication across the "newly enhanced mentorship team" around these issues. Occasionally a mentee decides to pursue research (or other scholarly activities) in a discipline that is not represented at their home institution. In this case, their effective "home-institution" mentor will help them enlist a "research mentor" at another institution while maintaining responsibility for the other elements of career development that are specific to the local policies and politics of their home base. Again, it's important that there is communication across this mentorship team to ensure there is not conflicting advice being given to the mentee.

- *Trustworthy*: Given the need for open communication, effective mentors must maintain the confidentiality of their mutual compact. Because mentees must be able to freely discuss problems with personal finances and academic advancement, their mentor should not directly control their academic appointment (mentors should be advocates here, not judges), base salary, or other substantial resources such as space or administrative support. Such controls interfere with the free and open exchange of ideas, priorities, aspirations, and criticisms.
- *Reliable*: Effective mentors keep mentoring appointments and follow through with their pledges. Accordingly, effective mentors don't take on new mentees unless they have the time to meet with them (and effective department chairs and deans don't take on more graduate students unless they also recruit the additional faculty required to mentor them!).
- *Actively listening*: In responding to their mentees, effective mentors exhibit all three steps of:
  - making sure they comprehend what their mentee is saying through both words and body language
  - making sure they retain what their mentee is communicating
  - making sure they avoid roadblocks that often interfere with communication (such as dismissing mentees' concerns or moralizing about them).
- *Motivating*: Effective mentors are role-models that *display* (not simply state!) their high motivation for academic excellence, ethical behavior, and proper professional conduct.
- *Self-appraising*: Effective mentors regularly evaluate their performance as a mentor through self-assessment and invited feedback from their mentees. Effective mentors periodically seek feedback (at least annually) about how

they are performing from their mentees, with an opportunity for a no-fault breakup if things aren't working. They must periodically evaluate their own performance, decide whether they remain the best person to mentor their mentee (and, if not, help find a more suitable mentor), and identify ways to improve their mentoring skills. As mentees progress, effective mentors also work with them on developing their own mentorship skills through role modeling and feedback.

Effective mentors' behaviors toward mentees

The foregoing personal attributes are expressed in specific behaviors toward their mentees:

- *Accessibility*, especially on short notice and for mentee emergencies; note that this doesn't have to be in-person but can be done over the phone, via Skype©, email etc.
- *Working hard to develop an important relationship with their mentee*, by working hard to make the mentor–mentee relationship a success. When differences in ethnicity, language, gender, and generation threaten the mentorship, effective mentors create safe, trusting, respectful, supporting partnerships that render these sometimes "undiscussable" issues discussable [5].
- *Consistently offering help in their mentee's best interests*, in defining and working toward their academic and personal goals. The foregoing two behaviors are expressed in the idea of mentors acting as "guides",

  > ... sensitive to the difference between a guide and somebody who forces the student into or the mentee into a particular path [who] may well offer some advice but recognize that it is only advice, it's not orders [7].

  Put another way: "The most important thing is not trying to solve their problems but to help them find solutions."
- *Identifying their mentee's current and potential strengths and weaknesses*. Through both experiences with prior mentees and the exercise of their understanding, honesty, active listening, and responsiveness, effective mentees identify, label, and help mentees recognize and build upon their current and potential strengths and overcome or avoid their weaknesses.
- *Assisting their mentees in defining and reaching their goals*. Two quotes from the qualitative assessment of the nomination letters received for the mentorship award at the University of California, San Francisco provide glowing examples of the previous two behaviors [2]:

  > As a mentor, [he] provided direction and opportunity, allowing me to chart my own path, but at the same time guiding me along the way.

[He] was like a solid rocket booster, ensuring that I achieved the lift and trajectory necessary to make it into orbit. But rather than dropping off at that point, he has remained a constant feature in my life, much like mission control, monitoring my progress, offering incredibly helpful advice on a regular basis, and serving as a sounding board, editor, or strategist, depending on what I needed.

- *Holding high standards for their mentee's achievements*: Demonstrated in another quote from the University of California, San Francisco report [2]:

  [He] continues to accurately assess my skills, knowledge, and attitudes, and to challenge me to seek higher personal achievement than I would on my own. So, [he] is an outstanding mentor because he saw what I could become.

- *Compatibility with their mentee's practice styles, visions, and personalities.* Effective mentors rapidly diagnose and compare their mentees' practice styles, visions, and personalities with their own, and quickly determine their compatibility. When there is a mismatch, effective mentors arrange for a more compatible mentor to take over.*

The professional stature of effective mentors
High professional stature is a cardinal requirement before becoming an effective mentor, for four reasons. First is the achievement of sufficient academic success and respect from one's peers for the mentor to be comfortable taking a back seat in matters of authorship, grants, and recognition of their mentee's work. Indeed, effective mentors actively pursue this secondary role. As we will describe in Chapter 5, disasters occur when mentors compete with their mentees for recognition. At its worst, it leads to the theft of mentee's ideas for mentor's grants and the embezzlement of lead authorships from mentees who earned them. Tragically, such competition is common [7], and mentees should seek help from chairs or program directors when this happens. Even when mentees regain their intellectual property and due recognition, they may be scarred by the experience, often have trouble trusting colleagues thereafter, and sometimes leave town. Moreover, we've observed two nasty effects on their junior colleagues who observe this awful behaviour. Worst, when it goes unchecked they may come to regard it as standard academic behavior and start modelling it themselves. Alternatively, they may regard it as a symptom of a second-rate institution and leave town, or leave academia altogether to avoid a similar experience.

---

* Note that through these actions, effective mentors also serve as role models for their mentees who (it is hoped!) will in turn become effective mentors.

The second reason why high professional stature is a prerequisite for effective mentors is their ability to call upon the networks of useful, helpful colleagues and contacts they established along the way in the academic, healthcare, research funding, and regulatory communities for the benefit of their mentees. Their ability to open doors to opportunities for social interaction, advice, electives and short-term secondments, more senior training posts, and even permanent academic posts can benefit both the quality and speed of their mentees' academic advancement.

The third reason why high professional stature is a prerequisite for effective mentoring is the mass of practical, pragmatic, time- and energy-saving strategies and tactics for conducting an academic career they already carry in their toolkits. They already know how to set and decide among competing priorities [8], protect writing time [9], manage email [10], say "no" (nicely) to requests to take on tasks that they really shouldn't [11], run an office, hire and manage staff, and the like. Mentees with access to these toolkits can take the enormous amounts of time and energy they save and devote them to academic pursuits and to improving their work–life balance.

The fourth reason is the "authority" that accompanies high professional status and can be used to shelter and rescue their mentees from the unreasonable demands and bad behavior of other, even senior, academics and administrators. When mentees are reluctant to say "no" (nicely) to requests to take on tasks that they really shouldn't, mentors can do it for them (or at least be identified as strongly advising against it). And senior mentors can come down like a ton of bricks on any "sharks" [12] who attempt to harm their mentees by word or deed.

Given the foregoing, although "peer mentors" [13, 14] – drawn from trainees or junior faculty with little or no more additional training or experience than their mentees – can provide excellent moral support and short-term practical advice, they lack the established academic success, networks, experience, and non-competitiveness of the effective mentors that are the focus of this chapter. The exception here, of course, are aging academics who, when seeking mentoring, look to their younger peers.

Effective mentees

The characteristics of effective mentees were identified in the University of California, San Francisco review of qualitative studies in mentorship discussed above, and are summarized in Table 2.2.

Table 2.2 Characteristics of effective mentees

Dimension	Characteristic
Personal attributes	Understanding/compassionate
	Enthusiastic
	Nonjudgmental
	Patient
	Honest
	Responsive
	Trustworthy
	Reliable
	Excels at active listening
	Open to feedback
	Self-appraising
Behaviors toward mentors	Takes responsibility for "driving the relationship"
	Respects meeting times
	Comes prepared
	Pro-active in identifying and presenting problems and issues
	Respectful of mentors' time and other commitments

Adapted from [7] Straus SE, Johnson MO, Marquez C, Feldman MD. Characteristics of successful and failed mentoring relationships: qualitative study across 2 institutions. Acad Med 2013; 88: 82–9 with permission from Wolters Kluwer Health.

Personal attributes of effective mentees
Mentees' personal attributes mirror those of effective mentors.
- *Understanding/compassionate*: Understanding "where their mentor is coming from," and deeply aware and sympathetic towards others' challenges and difficulties. For example, if their mentor is reviewing grant applications for several mentees who are working to the same deadline, effective mentees recognize and accommodate these multiple simultaneous demands.
- *Enthusiastic*: Like their mentors, effective mentees also display intense and eager enjoyment and interest in academic healthcare, in the pursuit of the research methods that will generate the new knowledge that will improve it, and in life in general. Enthusiastic mentees keep their mentors stimulated and also provide good role models for junior faculty and trainees.
- *Non-judgmental* about their mentor's values, attitudes and aspirations. While they might not agree with their mentor's ideas about "what is best" for their career paths and development, they will respect them as long as they don't inhibit or otherwise hamper the relationship. That being said, mentees sort out their own values, attitudes, and aspirations for themselves.
- *Patient* with their mentor's schedule, other commitments, and limitations.

- *Honest* in offering their ideas and opinions, in responding to criticisms, and in evaluating the success of the mentorship and how it might be improved (or, if necessary, terminated). When issues arise beyond the experience and competency of their mentors (e.g. parental leave brought to a childless mentor, conflicts with the on-call and on-service scheduling of a clinical department brought to a non-clinical mentor) they should not hesitate to ask for outside help.
- *Responsive* to any and all issues raised by their mentors.
- *Trustworthy* in maintaining the confidentiality of their mutual compact.
- *Reliable* in preparing for mentoring meetings, in keeping mentoring appointments, and in following through with pledges that they make to their mentor.
- *Actively listening*; in responding to their mentors, exhibiting all three steps of:
  - making sure they comprehend what their mentor is saying through both words and body language
  - making sure they retain what their mentor is communicating
  - making sure they avoid roadblocks that often interfere with communication (such as dismissing mentors' concerns or moralizing about them).
- *Open to feedback*: As one participant in a qualitative study of mentoring put it:

  > ...the mentee should listen to the mentor and take them seriously and that doesn't mean following every bit of advice...if you're working with someone and they're giving you advice you know if you kind of ignore all of it then it's sort of a fruitless interaction [7].

- *Self-appraising*, regularly evaluating their performance as budding academics through self-assessment and invited feedback from their mentor, teachers, junior trainees, and colleagues.

Effective mentees' behaviors toward mentors
- The University of California, San Francisco study identified the essential behavior of mentees taking responsibility for "driving the relationship":

  > ...you can't just go in and be an undifferentiated blob about what you want, you have to really have thought before you go in and meet with your mentor about what the issue is that you need help with and you know it's much more useful if you bring your own analysis in with you and then the mentor can give you their analysis and you can talk [7].

- Effective mentees respect meeting times with their mentors, come prepared with previously identified topics for discussion and timelines for projects, and are pro-active in identifying and presenting problems and issues.
- Effective mentees also follow through after meetings, carrying out the agreed tasks in a timely fashion. In doing so, they are respectful of the mentor's time and other commitments. This respect is expressed by sending drafts of manuscripts and grants [15, 16] in sufficient advance of meetings to permit mentors to give them thorough review; indeed, repeated requests for quick reviews without advance notice has been identified as a source of not only mentor stress and strained relations but, for mentors caring for multiple mentees, mentor burnout.

Productive mentoring

The foregoing attributes and behaviors of both mentors and mentees, when "in synch" and fully exercised, reveal themselves in the five benchmarks of productive mentoring, illustrated in Table 2.3:
- a *personal connection*, beyond friendship and far beyond the ordinary "pupil–teacher" fences
- a set of *shared values* around how one approaches research, clinical work, and social life
- mutual *respect* for each other's time, effort, and expectations
- *clear expectations* about accountability to each other
- *reciprocity* in both efforts and rewards.

Chapters 3 and 4 will show how these characteristics and behaviors can be harnessed into establishing, executing, and enjoying effective and efficient mentorships.

How many mentees can effective mentors mentor?

We identified 30 colleagues (listed in the Introduction) in North America, Europe, and Africa with track records for effectively mentoring graduate students and junior academics, and asked them this question. Here is our summary of their responses, stated in terms of the "prevalence" of mentees they were currently serving at the time of our survey.
1 At the graduate student/trainee level, they distinguished thesis supervision (which might be restricted to addressing the scientific issues involved in producing and defending a high-quality document) from mentoring for personal and professional career development.
2 Some of our colleagues supervise as many as six theses per year (and lament the end-of-term crush of simultaneous submissions and defenses).

Table 2.3 How the attributes and behaviors of mentors and mentees can result in positive "themes" in the mentoring process

Theme	Illustrations from qualitative interviews
Development of a *personal connection* between mentor and mentee	"… having that connection where you feel like someone actually cares to know what you're thinking and who you are and is really actually doing it because they care to rather than because you know they're forced to". "Mentors and mentees should have the 'same chemistry' but 'not just being friends". "There are many people that I did meet that had similar interests as me but there just wasn't a personal connection".
Shared values around their approach to research, clinical work, and personal life	"Mentorship worked when mentors were on a fairly common ground, have similar ideas and interests and values".
Mutual respect for one-another's time, effort, and qualifications	"Both individuals need to respect the qualifications of the other and the needs of the other and work together towards a common goal".
Clear expectations of the relationship, outlined at the outset and revisited over time, with both mentor and mentee held accountable to them	"Mutual accountability: not only that the mentor has expectations of the mentee, but that the mentee also has expectations of the mentor". "It's helpful to set up sort of those guidelines in the beginning, sort of what the mentee can expect from the relationship but also what the mentor expects you to know".
Reciprocity: recognizing the bidirectional nature of mentoring, including the consideration of strategies to make the relationship sustainable and mutually rewarding	"It's got to be a two way street – it can't just be a one way giving relationship 'cause then it's just going to burn out. I mean I think the mentor gets a lot out of just the satisfaction of seeing their mentee succeed and that is important onto itself, that's the most important part but you know beyond that the mentor also needs some sort of tangible reward from the relationship that will kind of refresh them and make them keep wanting to come back for more. And that can be you know being on a publication or being recognized".

Adapted from [7] Straus SE, Johnson MO, Marquez C, Feldman MD. Characteristics of successful and failed mentoring relationships: qualitative study across 2 institutions. Acad Med 2013; 88:82-9 with permission from Wolters Kluwer Health.

3 However, they rarely mentor more than three graduate students/trainees at a time (occasionally more than this at the MSc level, and usually fewer than this at the PhD level).

4 The number of mentees they are serving 'full-time' at the postgraduate/ junior faculty level exhibit two modes. Many mentors (especially those with heavy clinical responsibilities) work with just one mentee at a time (and often initiate this mentorship during their mentee's graduate

training), whereas the second cluster of mentors are serving three mentees at a time. Early on, this mentoring is intense, with weekly or even more frequent contact.

5   Mentoring intensity decreases as current mentees succeed in obtaining research grants and generate peer-reviewed publications, creating openings for new mentees.

6   However, academically successful mentees usually maintain links with their mentors, participating in periodic reviews of their progress and priorities, especially when considering job-opportunities.

7   The number of mentees reported above is an underestimate at centers where research associates, study coordinators, etc. also require mentoring.

The "human resource" implications of our survey results for departments and institutions who hope (or claim!) to provide high-quality mentoring for graduate students and new faculty are profound for all, and probably awesome for some. Short-term solutions include "mentoring at a distance" for some mentees' needs, but the creation or expansion of graduate programs in order to reap greater profit or prestige without the creation or expansion of high-quality mentoring capability deserve the resultant whirlwinds of student unrest and falling credibility. Similarly, if universities mandate that every faculty member has to have a mentor, they must also recruit, train, and maintain the additional mentors required to meet this goal, reimburse their additional travel requirements, and recognize their contributions in institutional promotion and tenure processes.

Gaps in the evidence

As we discussed, most of the material in this chapter is at a "moderate quality" GRADE level, based on cross-sectional surveys and interviews of mentors and mentees. We didn't find any literature looking at effective mentorship over an entire research career or for those in different career paths.

Bottom line and scenario resolutions

How well did your descriptions of the ideal attributes and behaviors of mentors and mentees match the ones described in the body of the chapter? If you missed important ones, think why. If we missed important ones, write to us at our website!

References

1. Sambunjak D, Straus SE, Marusic A. A systematic review of qualitative research on the meaning and characteristics of mentoring in academic medicine. Gen Intern Med 2010; 25: 72–8.

2. Cho CS, Ramanan RA, Feldman MD. Defining the ideal qualities of mentorship: A qualitative analysis of the characteristics of outstanding mentors. Am J Med 2011; 124: 453–8.

3. Romberg E, Mentoring the individual student: Qualities that distinguish between effective and ineffective advisors. J Dent Ed 1993; 57: 287–90.

4. Straus SE, Straus C, Tzanetos K. Career choice in academic medicine: a systematic review. J Gen Int Med 2006; 21: 1222–9.

5. Bickel J, Rosenthal SL. Difficult issues in mentoring: recommendations on making the "undiscussable" discussable. Acad Med 2011; 86: 1229–34.

6. Chittenden EH, Ritchie CS. Work–life balancing: challenges and strategies. J Palliat Med 2011; 14: 870–4.

7. Straus SE, Johnson MO, Marquez C, Feldman MD. Characteristics of successful and failed mentoring relationships: qualitative study across two institutions. Acad Med 2013; 88: 82–9.

8. Sackett DL. Clinician–trialist rounds. 3: Priority setting for academic success. Clin Trials J 2011; 8: 235–7.

9. Sackett DL. Clinician–trialist rounds. 1: Inauguration, and an introduction to time-management for survival. Clin Trials J 2010; 7: 749–51.

10. Oxman A, Sackett DL. Clinician–trialist rounds. 13. Ways to advance your career by saying "no" Part 1: Why to say "no" (nicely), and saying "no" to email. Clin Trials J 2012; 9: 806–8.

11. Oxman A, Sackett DL. Clinician–trialist rounds. 14 Ways to advance your career by saying "no" Part 2: When to say "no" and why. Clin Trials J 2013 (in press).

12. Johns RJ. How to swim with sharks: The advanced course. Trans Assoc Am Physicians 1975; 88: 44–54.

13. Santucci AL, Lingler JH. Schmidt KL *et al.* Peer-mentored research development meeting: a model for successful peer mentoring among junior level researchers. Acad Psych 2008; 32: 493–7.

14. Johnson KS, Hastings SN, Purser JL, Whitson HE. The junior faculty laboratory: an innovative model of peer mentoring. Acad Med 2011; 86: 1577–82.

15. Szatmari P, Sackett DL. Clinician–trialist rounds. 11. When your grant gets turned down – Part 1: Remorse, anger and reconciliation. Clin Trials J 2012; 9: 447–9.

16. Szatmari P, Sackett DL. Clinician–trialist rounds. 12. When your grant gets turned down – Part 2: Resurrection. Clin Trials J 2012; 9: 660–3.

Chapter 3 **How can you initiate mentorship?**

This chapter is written from the perspective of a mentee hoping to link to an effective mentor and establish an effective mentorship.

Scenario

You have finished postdoctoral training in clinical epidemiology after having already completed clinical training as a geriatrician. These were completed at different universities, and you have just been recruited to a faculty position at a third one where you have never previously worked. You have about 15 publications (with half of these from your graduate work and fellowship training and the other half from collaborative projects in which you are a co-author), and are working on an application for an operating grant and a salary support award; the latter requires a letter of support from a mentor. Your new chair is dynamic and appears supportive of your research niche. She encourages you to find a mentor right away. You don't know anyone at this new university but recognized your need to find a mentor who will not only guide you immediately in preparing your salary support award application, but will stick with you longer term to help you grow and succeed as a researcher, teacher, and clinician. How do you find a mentor?

How do you find a mentor?

In Chapter 2, we focused on what mentees should look for in a mentor and in this chapter, we'll build on this and discuss how to find a mentor and develop an effective mentoring relationship.

First, should you have to find a mentor on your own, or should you sit back and have one assigned to you?

Mentorship programs at some academic institutions assign mentors to mentees, and this assignment can be done by a department chair or a mentorship facilitator. Other programs leave it up to the mentees. This latter approach can work well for mentees already at a center for prior training, where they may already have identified their ideal mentor in a staff

Mentorship in Academic Medicine, First Edition. Sharon E. Straus and David L. Sackett.
© 2014 John Wiley & Sons, Ltd. Published 2014 by John Wiley & Sons, Ltd.

physician or faculty member with whom they worked on a clinical rotation or committee. But it can be a challenge for newcomers to that institution.

We haven't found any quantitative studies comparing the impact of assigned versus self-identified mentorship on the mentees. Four qualitative studies within a systematic review [1] explored mentee-initiated versus assigned mentorship (moderate-quality evidence) [2–5], and reported that mentees preferred to make the selection themselves. For example, in a qualitative study we conducted [3], mentees felt that being assigned a mentor could lead to "a forced relationship" that could lead to failure, and that "If you wouldn't do something with [your mentor] after work, then you probably are not going to be doing something with them at work either." Being assigned a mentor may ignore the interpersonal aspect of the relationship, which is crucial for effective mentorship. Although successful mentoring can develop through formal assignment, the relationship varies with the individuals involved and will succeed or fail depending on whether a personal connection is in place or can develop over time.

This is not to say that prospective mentees should be left entirely on their own in finding mentors. A couple of qualitative studies suggest that guidance for finding mentors is important (moderate-quality evidence) [1, 3]. For faculty members new to the institution, the studies found that it was particularly helpful to have guidance in finding a mentor. For example, the department chair could provide a list of potential mentors to the mentees based on similar interests. At University of California, San Francisco (UCSF), mentorship facilitators are available in each division, and they work with prospective mentees to identify potential mentors [6].

In our own work, some mentees have suggested an online matching system not unlike online dating strategies! For example, this strategy can match mentors and mentees based not only on their career interests, but also on leisure-time hobbies. We have not found any studies evaluating this type of strategy.

Sharon Straus has employed "speed mentoring" sessions in which mentees meet with several potential mentors in a single evening session, with appointments scheduled every 15 minutes [7]. This approach allows mentees to quickly identify both common interests and "chemistry," thereby narrowing their choices and determining whether they want to more deeply explore mentorship with a particular individual. Speed mentoring has been particularly effective when held in conjunction with national and international academic meetings, permitting prospective mentees to meet potential "distance-mentors" from outside their home institutions. Over the last five years, speed mentoring has been incorporated into our annual research training institute, and it consistently receives the highest participant-ratings of any event [7]. Cook and colleagues interviewed six mentors and seven mentees immediately after such a session, and all of them rated it as useful (but no data are available on what happened after these sessions) [8]. Another strategy is to use divisional meetings to identify and introduce potential mentors, followed by informal social events to facilitate meeting them (we even discovered that some divisions offer free coffee cards to prospective mentees and mentors to promote these informal meetings).

Regardless of how potential pairings are created, before formalizing the mentoring relationship, we recommend that mentees meet with their prospective mentor's prior mentees to elicit a "first-hand, second-opinion" of the mentor. These meetings can explore prior mentees' experiences, including examples of interactions that illustrate the mentor's personal qualities, breadth, time for mentoring, responses to emergencies, and so forth.*

Following on Chapter 2, we also found evidence on who shouldn't be a mentor. First, the mentor should not be someone with whom the mentee shares resources or who they depend on for resources (moderate-quality evidence) [1, 3, 9]. For example, the faculty member who determines the clinical schedule or allocates research or clinic space should not be the primary mentor for an individual who is competing for that space or for clinical protection. Second, when a trainee's graduate supervisor remains their primary mentor when they gain their faculty appointment, this can be perceived as the mentee's failure to develop their own unique and independent research niche [1, 3, 9]. Third, junior faculty may not have sufficient experience or expertise to be effective mentors [1, 3, 9]. Moreover, they may be more likely to "compete" with mentees if they are not yet firmly established in their own areas of research [1, 3, 9]. Finally, while it's not essential that the scientific methods mentor be from the same clinical discipline as the mentee,† it is important for the mentee have a career mentor

---

* After Sharon Straus meets with a potential mentee, she introduces them to other mentees with whom she's worked so that they can meet to explore whether there's a good fit. She finds this useful for three reasons: 1. They can meet with other mentees and start developing their own network of potential collaborators; 2. They can find out if they want to formalize the mentorship with her through discussions with the other mentees; 3. It allows both parties some time to think after the initial meeting and decide whether Sharon would be a "good fit" as mentor–mentee, avoiding pressure to make a commitment after a single meeting.

† Note that "scientific methods mentor" or "scientific mentor" can be used interchangeably and imply that the individual focuses on the research aspects of an individual's career. Similarly, we use the terms "academic mentor" and "career mentor" to refer to those mentors who provide advice on the overall career plan for the mentee.

from their own clinical discipline for guidance and advice on career progress, and around clinical and teaching responsibilities.

How should you structure your mentoring relationship?

Most mentorship studies consider the traditional mentorship approach of a single mentor linked to a single mentee (often called a *mentorship dyad*) [1, 9]. However, some studies have identified the potential for multiple mentors. For example, from the perspective of junior researchers interviewed in a large qualitative study (moderate-quality evidence), good mentoring meant having both an academic mentor (for guidance on promotion, career milestones, local politics, clinical work and work and life balance), and a scientific mentor (for guidance on research) [3]. Moreover, the mentees in this study felt that, while the academic mentor should be local, the scientific mentor could be from a distant site. Similarly, an individual mentee might need different mentors for clinical and teaching matters. Although such teams of mentors can provide useful and different perspectives to the mentee, we believe it's essential that communication be transparent across the team, to quickly identify and resolve occasions on which the mentee receives incompatible advice from different mentors.[‡]

Scientific methods mentorship at a distance may be necessary if the mentee works in a narrow field or at a small institution where there is no local mentor who has similar scholarly interests, or when such a mentor takes a post elsewhere and leaves this gap. Attending national or international meetings provides the opportunity to identify such distant mentors (see discussion in the previous section on speed mentoring), and research funders or home-department chairs should finance regular mentorship meetings between researchers with career development awards and their distant scientific methods mentors. In contrast, the qualitative literature suggests that career mentorship should be local, because it is important that the career mentor understands the local politics and institutional bureaucracy, as well as the local standards and criteria for promotion and tenure (moderate-quality evidence) [3, 10].

Can mentees' contemporaries – at their same stage of career development – provide sufficient mentoring? Evaluation of such "peer mentorship" is limited and possibly confounded [11, 12]. For example, Johnson and colleagues [12] described a peer-mentoring model for junior researchers at one institution, but there was no comparison group and

---

[‡] This knowledge exchange that can happen across a mentorship team also allows the mentors to learn from each other.

it is not clear how many of the mentees also had senior mentors. We conclude that although peer mentoring for junior faculty might be useful for "learning the lay of the land," problem solving day-to-day situations, and establishing and promoting collaboration, peer mentors obviously lack the experience and perspective that comes with greater academic and life-experience. Moreover, peer mentoring presents greater potential for competition between "mentee–mentor peers" if they are competing for the same pot of resources and the same early-investigator awards.

In contrast, peer mentoring can be quite helpful for more senior faculty, (and no alternative exists for the oldest!). Consider, for example, taking on a new job as dean of a medical school. This person would likely find it helpful to receive mentorship from a seasoned dean from another institution. However, given the lack of evidence on the effects and effectiveness of peer mentorship, for the remainder of this book we will focus our discussion on traditional mentorship offered by a senior to a junior colleague.

Should mentors and mentees be matched for gender, race or ethnicity? Qualitative studies (low-quality evidence) [3–5, 13, 14] reached mixed conclusions. Certainly, if a mentee wants gender matching with their mentor, this factor should be explicitly addressed, but it should be individualized. Indeed, in a recent study of otolaryngology residents, their least important characteristics for mentor matching were gender, race, or age [14]. Far more important was sensitivity to the unique needs of the mentee. For example, female faculty members who are considering children may benefit from mentorship from another woman around timing of parental leave or managing a career while raising a family [3, 15]. The experience of women in academic medicine has been perceived to be different from the experience of male colleagues and one study has suggested that female mentees may benefit from the advice of another woman which will reflect these different experiences [4].§ Discussion around issues of child care and parental leave might be topics for peer mentorship as well.

---

§ During one of the first mentorship meetings Sharon Straus had with Dave Sackett, he outlined what actions that he could fulfil, including assistance with career guidance and monitoring; He explicitly mentioned that since she was a woman they might have different experiences in academics and our personal lives and that if she wanted to obtain mentorship around when to have children and how to balance this with an academic career, he would facilitate linkage with a relevant female mentor. This proactive approach highlighted two things: 1. Mentors should individualize their approach to their mentees; 2. Mentors should facilitate connections with other mentors who can meet their mentee's needs as relevant. Interestingly, more recently we have had male mentees who wanted advice on parental leave and its impact on their careers and have referred them to appropriate mentors who could provide this guidance.

Matching of the mentor and mentee on race or ethnicity has also been postulated as a potential factor to consider [1]. However, there is very little evidence on this issue. Interestingly, in the qualitative study on mentorship that we completed at the University of Toronto and UCSF, one of the differences between these institutions was that many UCSF participants identified the need to consider matching based on ethnicity, whereas this issue was not mentioned at all by participants in multi-cultural Toronto (where English has become the minority language) [10].

Pairing mentors and mentees based on gender, race, and ethnicity may not be possible at institutions with small pools of otherwise appropriate mentors. This may be another situation where multiple mentors are required: one for scholarly matters and another matched for other needs of the mentee. This may also present an opportunity to explore mentorship at a distance for mentees' needs that are not served locally.

What should happen in the first meeting with your mentor?

Once a mentor has been identified, the initial meeting should occur in a safe, private, and welcoming environment; usually this is the mentor's office. While some mentorship programs encourage meeting for lunch or dinner, these venues might not ensure confidentiality. Regardless of its venue, the first session should establish and document the ground rules for the relationship, including:

- The format and content of the sessions:
  - The mentor and mentee should discuss the generation and pre-circulation of the agenda for their meetings, including how far in advance the mentor wants to receive this and what should be included.
  - They should also outline how they will prioritize topics at each meeting. For example, if the mentee prepares a list of topics often there may be more topics listed than could reasonably be covered in a one-hour meeting, requiring identification of key issues that need to be tackled in person and other that can be addressed via email after the meeting. Similarly, the mentor might have issues that they want to add to the list the mentee has prepared, and these should be prioritized as well.
  - Discussions should address in-person versus telephone versus email communication between the mentor and mentee. While in-person meetings are optimal, sometimes urgency and scheduling conflicts won't allow it, and sometimes the brevity of the agenda won't warrant it. In such cases, telephones and email can suffice.

- A proposed schedule for meetings:
  - The mentor and mentee should come to consensus on the duration and frequency of meetings. The initial meeting between the mentor and mentee will likely be far longer than subsequent meetings (we suggest scheduling them for 90 min). Subsequent meetings may be shorter but we find that longer meetings are necessary for discussing activities such as the mentee's annual review. The frequency of meetings between the mentor and mentee will depend on the needs of the mentee and should be adjusted to accommodate new and pressing issues.
- The accountability of both mentor and mentee to the success of the mentorship:
  - The mentor and mentee should discuss and come to agreement on their roles and their accountability for these roles. For example, they both should explicitly agree to mutual respect, open communication, listening to each other, and to sharing responsibility for the mentorship's success.
- The confidential nature of all discussions:
  - The mentor and mentee should explicitly discuss their approach to ensuring the confidential nature of all discussions; unless the relationship is seen to be secure and confidential, it will not promote open communication. Exceptions to this ground rule can occur by mutual consent (such as when it becomes necessary for the mentor to advocate on behalf of the mentee).
- A strategy for apportioning academic credit for any intellectual property that may arise from the mentorship:
  - It's useful to discuss the approach the pair will use for intellectual property around grants, publications, and other scholarly outputs. For example, they may use the initial meeting as an opportunity to discuss their approach to authorship of papers such as that outlined by the International Committee of Medical Journal Editors. We find it helpful to document this discussion so that it can be referred to, if needed, in future discussions.

We have found it useful for the mentee to prepare a summary in advance of this first meeting that includes:

- their current job description
- the time they have allocated to administration, education, research, clinical and other creative professional activities (and its validation in their contract or job description)
- their current activities
- their understanding of the requirements for advancement within the institution, including timelines

- their five lists as outlined in Chapter 4.1
- their short term (i.e. 1-year) goals and expected outcomes from achieving these goals
- their long term goals (e.g. 3–5 years) and expected outcomes from achieving these goals.

This mentee summary serves several functions:

1 It provides the mentee an opportunity to reflect on their current activities and their future goals in advance of the meeting.
2 It provides the mentor with an understanding of the mentee's job description and goals.
3 It can be used both to track progress on a regular basis and to perform "course corrections" if needed.

In our qualitative study [10], we found that some mentors used a checklist during this initial meeting to ensure that all important issues were addressed. We and others have discovered that a mentorship checklist is useful (as mentioned in Chapter 2), both at the initial meeting and at subsequent meetings. It is particularly useful in reminding mentors to consider all aspects of their mentee's career development and work/life balance, helping mentees reflect on the equilibrium (or lack thereof!) between their work and personal life. While discussions with mentees often focus on career issues, mentors should attend to how the mentee targets opportunities and ensure that they are not neglecting their personal life.[5] We give the checklist to our mentees so that they can set agendas and be prepared for each mentorship meeting.

We'll discuss the strategies and tactics employed in effective ongoing mentorships in Chapters 4.1–4.5.

Gaps in the evidence

As the reader has seen, there are substantial gaps in the evidence around optimal strategies for identifying appropriate mentors. Although we're not convinced that we'll ever see a proper randomized trial of assigned versus "discovered" mentors, cohort or case-control studies could at least determine

---

[5] Sometimes Sharon Straus finds that, in a one-hour meeting with a mentee, they spend so much time discussing their clinical activities and scholarly challenges that very little time is left for addressing their work/life balance. After trying different strategies to overcome this, the one that has proved most useful is for her to not only review the mentee's list of priorities for discussion, but also to reorganise their order so that work/life balance issues are discussed at the onset. This doesn't need to happen with every meeting, but regularly enough that we ensure that adequate time is given to these issues. This strategy also reinforces to the mentee that mentorship meetings are not just about scholarly work, and that we're interested and invested in their overall growth and development as an individual.

their differential impacts on productivity, promotion, and satisfaction. Similarly, we hope that quantitative studies will address the impact of various strategies for initiating mentorship, such as speed-mentoring sessions and informal social events.

Bottom line and scenario resolution

Returning to our scenario that opened this chapter:

1 You decide to meet with both the clinical division head and the director of research at your new institution, and ask them for a list of potential mentors who not only have similar scholarly interests to yours, but also have a track record in mentoring successful new investigators.
2 Ranking the entries on this list, you schedule meetings with your top choices and send them your CV in advance.
3 During this first interaction, you determine whether you have made a personal "connection" with them.
4 If so, you explore their approach to mentorship and decide whether it agrees with your own.
5 You use this first interaction to gauge their interest in providing you with mentorship.
6 If their interest is high, you ask them for introductions to some of their current and past mentees and arrange to meet with some of them.
7 When you meet with these other mentees you grill them about their mentoring experience, the challenges they face within their mentorship, and their mentor's approach to mentorship, including time availability and strategies for communication.
8 You synthesize all the foregoing information, select the best potential mentor for you, and arrange a second meeting to confirm their interest.
9 To your mutual delight, they agree.
10 During your first formal session with them (which happens within the first month of your appointment) you prepare both of you in advance by generating and forwarding (a week in advance) a summary document that includes your job description, your current activities, and both your short- and long-term goals.
11 You also prepare and forward a prioritized list of topics you'd like to address at that first session, including a new research project you would like their advice around, and an educational request from your division head to develop a series of sessions for educating postgraduate residents on geriatric medicine.

References

1. Sambunjak D. Straus SE. Marusic A. A systematic review of qualitative research of the meaning and characteristics of mentoring in academic medicine. J Gen Int Med 2010; 25: 72–8.

2. Jackson VA, Palepu A, Szalacha L *et al*. "Having the right chemistry": a qualitative study of mentoring in academic medicine. Acad Med 2003; 78: 328–34.

3. Straus SE, Chatur F, Taylor M. Issues in the mentor-mentee relationship in academic medicine: qualitative study. Acad Med. 2009; 84: 135–9.

4. Koopman RJ, Thiedke CC. Views of family medicine department chairs about mentoring junior faculty. Med Teach 2005; 27: 734–7.

5. Williams LL, Levine JB, Malhotra S, Holtzheimer P. The good-enough mentoring relationship. Acad Psychiatry 2004; 28: 111–5.

6. Johnson MO, Subak LL, Brown JS *et al*. An innovative program to train health services researchers to be effective clinical and translational research mentors. Acad Med 2010; 85: 484–9.

7. Straus SE, Brouwers M, Johnson D *et al*. Core competencies in the science and practice of knowledge translation: description of a Canadian strategic training initiative. Implement Sci 2011; 6: 127.

8. Cook DA, Bahn RS, Menaker R. Speed mentoring: an innovative method to facilitate mentoring relationships. Med Teacher 2010; 32: 692–4.

9. Sambunjak D, Straus SE, Marusic A. Mentoring in academic medicine: a systematic review. JAMA 2006; 296; 1103–15.

10. Straus SE, Johnson MO, Marquez C, Feldman M. Characteristics of successful and failed mentoring relationships: qualitative study across two institutions. Acad Med 2013; 88: 82–9.

11. Santucci AL, Lingler JH. Schmidt KL *et al*. Peer-mentored research development meeting: a model for successful peer mentoring among junior level researchers. Acad Psych 2008; 32: 493–7.

12. Johnson KS, Hastings SN, Purser JL, Whitson HE. The junior faculty laboratory: an innovative model of peer mentoring. Acad Med 2011; 86: 1577–82.

13. Chung KC, Song JW, Kim HM *et al*. Predictors of job satisfaction among academic faculty members: Do institutional and clinical staff differ? Med Ed 2010; 44: 985–5.

14. Gurgel RK, Schiff BA, Flint JA *et al*. Mentoring in otolaryngology training programs. Otolaryngology Head Neck Surg 2010; 142: 487–92.

15. Leslie K, Lingard L, Whyte S. Junior faculty experiences with informal mentoring. Med Teach 2005; 27: 693–8.

Chapter 4.1 Some effective mentoring strategies and tactics

Part 1: Mentorship meetings, priority setting, and time management

The characteristics and behaviors of effective mentors and mentees presented in Chapter 2 provide an enormous opportunity for both parties to achieve not only academic success but also personal fulfillment. But this opportunity, by itself, is not enough to achieve these goals. Both parties have to seize it and execute some specific strategies and tactics that are essential to this success and fulfillment. The objective of this chapter is to begin to identify these strategies and tactics and describe their application.*

Scenario

You are part of a brand new mentor–mentee pair, and are both excited and apprehensive as you approach your first mentoring session. There are so many matters you could address at this initial session that you're not quite sure where to start – should it focus on education, teaching, research ideas, research grants, start-up funds, writing, career plans, promotion, finances, space, equipment, travel, recreation, family-time, or any other of the myriad nuts and bolts that have to come together to create academic and personal success? How should the two of you organize this new mentorship so that it becomes capable of addressing all these issues in an effective, orderly fashion that also responds quickly to academic and personal emergencies?

We found no randomized trials that validated the strategies and tactics described here. Rather, they are a distillate of our personal experiences as mentees and mentors, of our systematic literature reviews, of our qualitative research among both mentees and mentors, and of our "colleague survey" of 44 colleagues around the world. Accordingly, the evidence in this chapter meets the moderate-quality criterion of the GRADE Working Group.[†]

---

* Many of them have appeared previously as "Clinician-trialist rounds" in the journal *Clinical Trials*, and will be cited as they arise here.
[†] See http://www.gradeworkinggroup.org/

Mentorship in Academic Medicine, First Edition. Sharon E. Straus and David L. Sackett.
© 2014 John Wiley & Sons, Ltd. Published 2014 by John Wiley & Sons, Ltd.

The top-ranked strategies emerging from these sources were:
- holding regular meetings (with pre-agreed agendas)
- establishing mentees' academic and social priorities and the time-management tactics required to meet and balance them
- protecting mentees from the myriad "dys-opportunities" they will encounter along the way.

The first two of these strategies will be explored in this chapter, the third in the following chapter, and additional strategies will appear in the subsequent three chapters.

Strategy 1: Holding regular meetings, with pre-agreed agendas

Our colleague survey urged us to recommend frequent (weekly at the start) meetings, preceded by a mentee-prepared agenda (in sufficient time for the mentor to digest) and followed closely by a set of minutes describing agreed-upon tasks for both members, with mutually-agreed deadlines for their completion. In addition, mentors like Sharon Straus – after the mentee's agenda is addressed – follow-up with items from a checklist such as that in Box 4.1.1 to be sure that all relevant mentoring issues are addressed. Moreover, some mentors are so concerned that social and financial issues ("are you okay and having fun?") receive proper attention that they explore these domains even before attending to the agenda.

Box 4.1.1 Mentorship checklist

Overall goals are to: advise, provide resources, provide opportunities, protect.
1 Assess the mentee
  a) Check in
  b) Assess for any urgent issues
2 Review their pre-circulated agenda
  a) Review pending items
    i. Administration
      - hospital
      - university
      - provincial
      - national
      - international
    ii. Clinical
      - inpatient
      - outpatient
      - on call responsibilities

---

    iii. Research
- publications
- grants
- presentations
- grant review panels

    iv. Teaching/training/providing mentoring
- undergraduate
- postgraduate
- graduate
- continuing education

    v. Creative professional activity
- Specify i.e. tool development for patients, clinicians

    vi. Work–life balance

    vii. Career guidance
- review individual development plan and CV

  b) Assess the time available for this session

  c) Prioritize the agenda accordingly (and how you might handle some of it by email or telephone)

3 Assist/advise

  a) Ask clarifying questions

  b) Set clear and measurable goals

  c) Give advice and suggest resources

  d) Agree on timeline for deliverables

4 Provide opportunities

  a) Consider potential collaborations/projects

5 Advocate/protect

  a) Identify shark attacks and determine what actions are needed and who will execute them

6 Wrap up

  a) Clarify expectations of mentor and mentee

  b) Schedule the next meeting

Meeting places must be private locations where mentees feel comfortable and secure, and meeting contents and minutes must remain strictly confidential. If mentors' or mentees' offices fail the former criteria, alternative venues must be negotiated.

Subsequent meetings are held as often as desired or required (as for emergencies), and always for a pre-specified purpose. They can be conducted in person, via Skype© or its alternatives, or over the phone, with email exchanges along the way. As mentoring proceeds, the agenda begins to include items around the evaluation of both members' performance (are both of them sticking to their ends of the bargain?) and the mentorship itself.

Strategy 2: Establishing mentees' academic and social priorities and the time-management tactics required to meet and balance them

Our colleague survey labeled this the primary function of the mentorship, and the chief determinate, not only of its success, but of the academic and social success of the mentee. We agree with their conclusion and with its determinants: the tactics of periodic priority setting and rigorous time management.

The tactic of periodic priority setting

Academics soon discover that, if they don't set the priorities for what they do, someone else (especially their clinical and academic bosses) will. The tactic for avoiding this is the setting down, monitoring, periodically reviewing (with one's mentor), and updating of one's personal career priority lists. This tactic, though trivially simple in format, is dreadfully difficult in execution, yet vital to both career success and happiness.

The approach applied by the authors and several members of our colleague-survey cohort urges mentees to generate four lists [1]:

- List #1: Things mentees are doing now that they want to *quit*.
- List #1a: Things that mentees have just been asked to do that they want to *refuse* to do.
- List #2: Things mentees are not doing that they want to *start* doing.
- List #3: Things mentees are doing that they want to *continue* doing.
- List #4: Strategies *to improve the balance* within these lists by shortening Lists #1 and #1a (*quit* and *refuse*) and lengthening List #2 (*start*) over the next six months.

Note that the entries on this list are about *doing* (things like research, clinical practice, teaching, writing, and the like). They are not about *having* (things like space, titles, rank, or income). Note, too, that there is no "cop-out" list for "things mentees *have* to do." Have-to-do tasks must be thought through until they can be allocated to either List #1 (*quit*) or List #3 (*continue*).

Mentees can generate Lists #1 (*quit*) and #3 (*continue*) by reviewing their diaries, grants, and publications for the period since their last update.[‡] List #1a (*refuse*) is generated from their current stack of requests from bosses and colleagues who are attempting to transfer problems and jobs from their desks to the mentee's.

[‡] Note that with the use of electronic annual activity reports at many institutions, this tool (which should be updated regularly and not just annually, so the task is less onerous) can be used to easily assess activities for list generation.

List #2 (*start*) should be the most exciting one. Mentees can create it from many and different sources:

- the next research question that logically follows the answer to their last one
- the ideas that arise from their clinical and educational triumphs, failures, questions, and conundrums that inevitably attend the thoughtful care of patients
- the brainstorms that occur while reading, sleeping, driving, or during conversations with colleagues
- the ideas that are formed during trips to meetings or other research centers
- the inspirations that arise in reading other people's research in depth and with a critical eye
- long-held aspirations that are now within reach
- job offers
- changes in their life goals or personal relationships
- the desire to try their hand at administration
- etc.

Contemplating the length and content of List #3 (*continue*) enables self-diagnosis and insight. If it's long, is it comfortable but complacent, stifling further growth? Worse yet, is it the list of an expert, comprising the tasks required to protect and extend mentees' personal "turf" in ways that are leading them to commit the "sins of expertness?" [2].

The next, crucial step is to titrate Lists #2 (*start*) and #3 (*continue*) against Lists #1 and #1a (*quit* and *refuse*). Academic and personal disaster results from the imbalance between what mentees are doing and what is expected of them. This imbalance is inevitable when mentees fail to avoid doing enough things on Lists #1 and #1a (*quit* and *refuse*) to make it possible to pursue List #2 (*start*), while continuing things on List #3 (*continue*).

For "time-imbalanced" academics, there are two outcomes. First, mentees can work day and night, keep up, and trade their family, friends, and emotional well-being for a reputation as a world-class academician. Second, regardless of whether they work day and night, mentees can fall behind and gain reputations as a 'non-finishers.' Either way, they increase their risk of slipping into that emotional exhaustion, cynicism, feeling clinically ineffective, and developing a sense of depersonalization in dealing with patients, colleagues, and family known as "burn-out." [3].

Making and updating lists have two goals, then. One is the prevention of burn-out. The other is the realization of a set of research, teaching, and clinical activities that makes it fun for mentees to go to work.

All the foregoing tasks lead to List #4, a tactical plan for *improving the balance* within mentees' lists by terminating entries in Lists #1 and #1a (*quit* and *refuse*) and creating time for Lists #2 and #3 (*start* and *continue*).

On the one hand, mentees will add greatly to their academic reputations when their List #4 (*improving the balance*) advocates gradual and orderly change through evolution, such as giving six months' notice on List #1 (*quit*) entries and by helping to find and train their successor. Along the way, they can gain administrative skills by sorting out which of the List #1 (*quit*) tasks can be delegated to their assistants, with what degrees of supervision and independence. On the other hand, mentees will damage their reputations if their List #4 (*improving the balance*) calls for revolution, precipitous resignation, or running away.

To illustrate the foregoing (and to emphasize the career-long benefits of creating these lists), Table 4.1.1 contains excerpts from a recent periodic priority list created by Sharon Straus.

Mentees can start making and updating priority lists as soon as they gain the smallest degree of control over their day-to-day activities and destiny. Rather than wait until they take up their first faculty appointments or defend their theses, we suggest that they begin making them as soon as they start their graduate training, using their mentor's priority list as an example if necessary. We recommend reviewing and updating these lists at least every six months, and more often if needed. Their discussion and evaluation ought to be a key periodic element of meetings with their mentors.

The tactic of time management

The successful execution of this tactic begins with mentees acknowledging the only barrier that they can never overcome: the number of hours in a day. Somehow it needs to be managed within five domains: performing research, writing for publication, caring for patients, teaching, and the mentee's social and family life. Every mentor's vital functions include helping mentees develop, apply, and monitor tactics for time management. Setting aside sufficient time for the first and last of these domains cannot occur without strictly controlling the middle three, and we will begin with them.

Time management and writing for publication

The most important element of time-management for the academic success of individuals in a 'research' faculty stream is setting aside and ruthlessly protecting time that is spent writing for publication [4, 5]. Indeed, for some successful academic clinicians, the only control over their schedule has been protected writing time. Conversely, very few academic clinicians will succeed without protecting their writing time, regardless of how well they control the other elements of their schedules. For some, this protected writing time occurs outside normal working hours, but the price of such nocturnal and weekend toil is often paid by family and friends, and is a set-up for burn-out.

Table 4.1.1   Excerpts from Sharon's 2012 priority list

List #1   Things I'm doing now that I want to *quit*:
  1   3 committees on which I currently serve which are not aligned with my academic interests
  2   Associate editor for a journal – time on someone else's ms. rather than mine!

List #1a   Things I've just been asked to do that I want to *refuse* to do:
  3   4 invitations to review mss. for various journals
  4   Join 3 committees (local, provincial) and 2 grant review committees
  5   Mentor 2 new faculty members – I don't think I have the time to meet their needs
  6   Respond to a journalist's request for a comment on someone else's article
  7   5 requests to review grants for others

List #2   Things I'm not doing that I want to *start* doing:
  8   Spend more time with my research team
  9   Work on research to optimize prioritization of management issues in patients with multiple chronic diseases
  10   Write an editorial on the risks of partnering with industry to develop strategies to implement guidelines
  11   Develop a decision aid for patients/families with MCI and AD who are considering cognitive enhancers
  12   Develop and evaluate the impact of novel formats for systematic reviews to enhance their use and readability by clinicians, patients, and policy makers

List #3   Things I'm doing that I want to *keep* doing:
  13   Working on the next editions of our EBM textbook and our KT book
  14   Working on the first edition of our mentorship textbook
  15   Mentoring
  16   Supervising graduate students
  17   Writing manuscripts (in a timely fashion) for relevant journals
  18   Improving uptake of my research (and those of others) through developing and evaluating implementation interventions targeting patients and clinicians
  19   Conducting systematic reviews/meta-analysis of relevant clinical questions
  20   Exploring the methods of conducting systematic reviews of complex interventions
  21   Attending on the inpatient services
  22   Developing capacity building network in implementation with colleagues internationally (e.g. GREAT network)
  23   Developing our consultation service in implementation for researchers, clinicians, managers
  24   Supervising, having fun with my research/consultation team
  25   Attending relevant divisional meetings
  26   Working as associate editor on 1 journal
  27   Examining for the Royal College internal medicine exams
  28   Protecting time for family and friends

List #4   Strategies for *improving the balance* within my lists by shortening Lists #1 and #1a (*quit* and *refuse*) and lengthening List #2 (*start*) over the next 6 months:
  29   Resign from committees
  30   Implement a 24–48-h rule – don't say yes to any more article reviews or committees unless think about it for 48 h and review priority list!!

The prototypically successful academic clinician sets aside one day per week for this activity (except during periods of intensive clinical responsibilities, to be discussed in a following paragraph), and clearly means it by telling everyone that they aren't available for chats, phone calls, email, committees, classes, or departmental meetings that day.

Academic writing is almost never easy,[§] although many find it nonetheless enormously enjoyable and gratifying. Given the difficulty of writing well, no wonder so many academics find other things to do when they should be writing for publication. The great enemy here is procrastination (which has been exacerbated by the pervasive nature of email and more recently, Twitter), and mentors play a vital role in helping mentees establish rigorous, self-imposed rules for their protected writing time. It is:

- *not* for writing grants
- *not* for refereeing manuscripts from other academics (aren't they already ahead of the mentee with their writing?)
- *not* for answering electronic or snail mail or any other social media
- *not* for keeping up with the literature
- *not* for responding to non-emergencies that can wait until day's end
- *not* for making lists of what should be written about in the future
- *not* for merely outlining a paper
- *not* for coffee-breaks with colleagues.

Early on, self-imposed daily quotas of intelligible prose may be necessary, and these should be set at realistic and achievable levels (as small as 300 coherent words for beginners). It is imperative that no interruptions occur on writing days. Unless mentees are protected by ruthless assistants and respected by garrulous colleagues, this often can best be achieved by creating a writing room away from the office; whether this is elsewhere in the building or at home depends on distractions (and family obligations) at these other sites. Writing in a separate, designated room permits mentees to create stacks of drafts, references, and the other organized litter that accompanies writing for publication. It also avoids their unanswered mail, unrefereed manuscripts, undictated patient charts, and the other distracting, disorganized litter of a principal office. Moreover, if email is disabled in the computer in their writing room (and their Blackberry is hidden from sight and sound), a major cause for procrastination is avoided.

Mondays hold three distinct advantages as writing days for academic clinicians who are not on call. First, the non-clinical things that "can't wait" are much more likely to arise on Fridays, and very few things that arise over the weekend can't wait until Monday night or Tuesday. Second, a draft that

---

[§] . . . and people who deny this are either liars or awful writers!

gets off to a good start on Monday often can be completed during brief bits of free time over the next four days and sent out for comments by week's end. Third, the comforting knowledge on a Sunday night that Monday will be protected for writing can go far in improving and maintaining mentees' mental health, family function, and satisfaction as aspiring academics. And, of course, the more of their colleagues who write on the same day each week (except when on the clinical service), the greater the opportunity for trading offices and the lesser the conflicts in scheduling meetings.

Time management and clinical activities

The second important element of time-management addresses how aspiring academic clinicians schedule their clinical activities [6]. On the one hand, they want to maximize the delivery of high-quality care and high-quality clinical teaching. On the other hand, they need to avoid, or at least minimize, conflicts with the other elements of their academic careers.

Of course, their clinical work should complement their research. Indeed, clinical observations, frustrations and failures should be a major source of the questions they pose in their research. But both activities require adequate blocks of a mentee's full attention. Having to switch back and forth between them several times a week is a recipe for frustration and failure.

Many successful academic clinicians from inpatient disciplines solve this by devoting specific blocks (of, say, one month) of on-service time to focus on clinical service and teaching. When on service, their total attention can be paid to the needs of their patients and clinical learners. Little or no time is spent writing, travelling, attending meetings, or teaching non-clinical topics (when house staff and students are occupied elsewhere over noon hours, these can sometimes be devoted to catching up with other tasks). This total devotion to clinical activities often will permit them to take on more night call and a greater number of patients and clinical learners. (During each month "on" his medical inpatient service at Oxford, Dave Sackett took call 10 times, and his clinical team of up to 16 learners and visitors admitted about 230 patients. Moreover, in addition to their individual daily bedside teaching rounds, Dave and his fellows provided over 50 hours of extra, learner-level clinical teaching during their month "on service.")

When off service, however, mentees' time and attention should shift as completely as possible to research and non-clinical teaching. Ideally, they should have no night call when they are off service. Moreover, they need not routinely see every discharged patient at a post-hospital outpatient follow-up visit (by 'phoning his patients' general practitioners within 48 hours after admission and again within 48 hours before discharge, Dave reduced his out-patient follow-ups by >95%).

If mentees are worried about getting rusty or out of date between their months on service, they might elect to shadow the rounding teams on relevant services for a week just before reassuming command. Surgeons coming off a period of full-time research may want to "warm-up" by assisting at a few relevant operations before taking over.

Like so many other elements of academic success, this sort of time-management is fostered by the development of a team of like-minded individuals who spell one another in providing excellent clinical care. A survey of physicians in their second decade of clinical practice suggested that there needs to be at least three like-minded clinicians to make this strategy work [7].

Clinicians in other fields (e.g. intensive care and some of the surgical specialities) may find it preferable to allocate time to inpatient clinical practice in units of one week. Another variant of scheduling is practiced by clinicians whose incomes are derived solely from private practice. Some of them devote three weeks each month to intensive clinical practice, followed by a "free" fourth week devoted entirely to their highly successful applied research programmes.

This still leaves mentees with the outpatient dilemma. Academic clinicians typically accept ambulatory referrals to their general or subspecialty clinics one or two half days every week. But in addition to the time spent during the clinic session itself, they soon learn that they have to spend several hours during the following two to three days chasing down lab results, talking with referring clinicians, obtaining collateral information from family/caregivers, and dictating notes. This additional time interrupts and often disrupts their research, teaching, and travel, diminishing their research and writing productivity, peace-of-mind, and fun. Moreover, this pattern of weekly clinics may even lower the quality of patient care. What happens when a mentee is 1000 km away when their out-patient gets sick during the diagnostic tests they've ordered, or has an adverse reaction after starting a new medication?

A solution mentees ought to at least consider is to replace their weekly out-patient sessions with a single monthly concentration of all four into two days of back-to-back-to-back-to-back clinics. By staying in town for the few days following this out-patient "blitz," they can tie up four clinics' loose ends all at once (especially if they can delegate chasing down lab results) and the rest of their month is free for academic activities. Unfortunately this strategy often isn't feasible for primary care clinicians; they might, however, be able to schedule their clinics on the same one to two days each week and stick to it.

Time management and teaching

This section is for mentees whose major career focus is health research; academic clinicians whose major focus is education obviously will devote the majority of their time to that endeavor [6].

For academic clinicians with a major focus on health research, one of the sadder realities of pursuing a primary research career is to be forced to consider teaching commitments under the heading of time management. Of course the opportunities and requests for teaching are endless, and the worthiness and fun of teaching are huge. That's why some universities have started to recruit and support clinician-scientists who focus on education research. However, unless mentees are education-researchers, most universities offer tiny (or even negative) rewards for their teaching efforts and accomplishments. Rather, their promotion and tenure remain dominated by first-authored publications in high-impact journals. Put quite simply, the time they spend teaching is time taken away from performing and (especially) from publishing their research. No wonder, then, that so many clinical research institutes boast that their recruits need not do any teaching. And, no wonder that mentors and those who oversee career investigator awards caution mentees against spending "too much time" teaching.

Accordingly, mentors may want to explore the following issues and tactics with their academic research mentees:

1 Examine your university's teaching requirements (if any) for promotion and tenure and be sure your mentee meets them. But help them focus their teaching so that it helps, not hinders, their career development. For example, undergraduate education may include supervision of undergraduates conducting research projects. And be sure that mentees maintain their "teaching portfolios" (with whatever syllabi, time records, evaluations, recognitions, etc. that your university requires). This portfolio should be started when still a graduate student to ensure that good documentation is kept. There is nothing worse than being asked to provide evidence of teaching and having to recreate it. Finally, mentors can help mentees organize their CVs and update them whenever appropriate. For example, we encourage our mentees to keep everything – any email, note, or evaluation – from any learner commenting on an educational session or interaction. These materials can provide strong support for promotion and tenure.

2 During their months on the inpatient clinical service (when they're not writing anyway), mentees can be encouraged to spend huge amounts of time teaching clinical skills/therapeutics/clinical physiology/evidence-based medicine at the bedside, so that they earn reputations as outstanding

clinical teachers. This is an area where clinician-mentors can make major contributions by "modelling" effective bedside teaching.

3 Mentees can be advised not to go on service when there are no students and house staff to teach, and to avoid clinical teaching when they are off service.

4 Mentors who teach research methods can invite their mentees to become junior co-tutors with them. In these roles, mentees not only earn teaching credits, but also can consolidate their own methodological learning while they pick up useful teaching strategies and tactics from a seasoned senior colleague.

5 Mentees should be advised to avoid the energy sink of taking responsibility for organizing or running an entire course early in their careers. Similarly, graduate student supervision should be taken on cautiously at career onset – we encourage people to join a thesis committee first before taking on the responsibility of graduate student supervision. (Avoiding this and myriad other "dys-opportunities" is the focus of Chapter 4.2.)

6 Finally, mentees should be discouraged from teaching on their writing days.

Time-management and social–family priorities

Everyone has to figure out what the appropriate work–life balance is for him or her. It's very easy to get caught up in our academic productivity and spend each summer and holiday period working on the next grant deadline or manuscript. And this behaviour often gets positively reinforced by colleagues and department heads (comments like: "XX always answers email quickly, even on the weekends" or "We need more people like YY who brings in several grants each year"). However, work is only a small part of our life overall.

Here are some useful strategies we've found helpful for our mentees to consider as they try to improve their work–life balance:

1 Hire a dog walker/cook/personal concierge/cleaning person etc. to do all of the activities that you don't like doing so that you can spend the time on things that you like to do. We have several friends and colleagues who retained their children's nanny after the children had grown because the nanny did many of the jobs that allowed them to have some free time to spend with family and friends.

2 Avoid committees that are known to meet at 7:30 am when you have small children. Many of these meetings times are set by people who don't have the responsibility of getting their kids ready for school and we suggest these be boycotted unless you're able to find childcare easily during this

time. Along the same line, you shouldn't schedule meetings for early in the mornings or late in the evenings, so you can role model this behaviour to others.

3 Take advantage of parental leave and ensure that work doesn't creep into it. We see so many people who take parental leave but are continuing to work, albeit from home, almost full time. It's useful to plan which parent will take time off and when, to optimise the leave.

4 Schedule regular social occasions with family and friends as rigorously as you schedule academic appointments. It sounds strange that academics have to schedule time for social occasions, but we often find that friends and colleagues (and ourselves!) get caught up in academic deadline after deadline and only later realise that their friendships, family relationships, and hobbies have fallen by the wayside through neglect.

5 Develop a strategy for answering email when on holiday. You could put an "away" message on your email to let people know that you will respond to them when you return. Because this can lead to a backlog with hundreds of emails on your return, some academics employ an "away" message that asks senders to repeat their message after you return if they are still relevant. Still others find it less stressful to continue to follow their email daily when on holiday – so again, find what works for you but make sure you're not spending all of your downtime on work email. See Chapter 4.2 for more strategies and tactics for handling email.

We close with some special considerations for mentors:

1 Mentees who are single parents have additional challenges and may not have the funds available to hire additional help. Strategies that could be considered include linking with others who might want to share the hiring of nannies/house cleaners.

2 When meeting with mentees, routinely ask about work–life balance and find out when they last did something fun outside of work. If we notice a pattern in which they're not doing anything outside of work, encourage them to schedule a "fun night/day/weekend" and ask them to report to us on what they did. Also, as mentors, we need to role model this behaviour for our mentees to show that we're also doing things outside of work – we've found that mentees find it useful to see how we achieve balance in our own lives. However, this is also an opportunity to point out that each of us has to find the right balance for our own situation.

3 We need to vigorously promote a culture that doesn't devalue people whose academic productivity is reduced when they take parental leave or time off to look after a sick parent. There remains a stigma in academics

attached to these "gaps in the CVs" that we must alleviate through promoting policies that facilitate such absences.

Bottom line and scenario resolution

1 Mentee: Ten days before your first meeting, you email your mentor with the entire list of all your questions, priorities, doubts, fears, and suggestions for how the mentorship might best help you address them.

2 Mentor: You email back at once, thanking your mentee for the list, and suggesting that they rank-order its contents by urgency. You enclose a copy of the Box 4.1.1: "Mentoring meeting checklist", both to show "where I'm coming from" and as a starting point for negotiating how the two of you want to run your meetings.

3 Mentee: Modifying the Box 4.1.1 template to suit, you slot the items on your list into it and email it back, apologizing for sending it the night before you meet.

4 Both: Your initial mentoring meeting goes wonderfully well. You trade bios and interests, laugh at each other's jokes, put each other at ease, work your way through the mentoring meeting checklist, and by the end of the session you both are becoming comfortable expressing feelings, opinions, and even disagreements.

5 Both: Through this progressively easier give-and-take, you modify the mentoring meeting checklist until it fits you both, and agree to use it for future meetings.

6 Mentee: You make a good start through your list of questions, are swiftly helped to confront the fact that it contains far more challenges, opportunities, and tasks than you can take on all at once, and realize that you have to either "prioritize" or drown.

7 Mentor: You hand your mentee a reprint of reference [1] on priority setting for academic success, suggest that they study it to see if it might be helpful, and – if so – put it on the agenda for your next mentoring meeting.

8 Both: You agree on a time and place for your next meeting, and on a deadline for submitting its agenda in sufficient advance that it can receive proper attention before you meet.

9 Mentee: You prepare a brief summary of the meeting and copy it to your mentor.

10 Mentor: You review the summary, add comments and suggestions, and copy it back to your mentee, adding a note that, from your perspective, you think the mentorship is off to an excellent start.

11 Mentee: You respond with an email of agreement and appreciation for the great start.

References

1. Sackett DL. Clinician-trialist rounds: 3. Priority setting for academic success. Clin Trials J 2011; 8: 235–7.
2. Sackett DL. The sins of expertness and a proposal for redemption. BMJ 2000; 320: 1283.
3. Shanafelt TD, Boone S, Tan L, *et al*. Burnout and satisfaction with work-life balance among US physicians relative to the general US population. Arch Intern Med. 2012; 172: 1377–1385.
4. Sackett DL. Clinician-trialist rounds. 1: Inauguration, and an introduction to time-management for survival. Clin Trials J 2010; 7: 749–51.
5. Reidenberg MM. Issues in developing the medical scientist, Part 3: Evaluation of scientific achievement. J Investigative Med 2004; 52: 361–3.
6. Sackett DL. Clinician-trialist rounds: 2. Time-management of your clinical practice and teaching. Clin Trials J 2011; 8: 112–4.
7. Spears BW. A time management system for preventing physician impairment. J Fam Pract 1981; 13: 75–80.

Chapter 4.2 Some effective mentoring strategies and tactics

Part 2: Protecting mentees from "dys-opportunities"

In the previous chapter we described how our personal experiences as mentees and mentors, our systematic literature reviews, our qualitative research among both mentees and mentors, and two independent surveys of colleagues around the world identified three vital strategies that mentors ought to execute in serving their mentees:

- holding regular meetings (with pre-agreed agendas)
- establishing mentees' academic and social priorities and the time-management tactics required to meet and balance them
- protecting mentees from the myriad "dys-opportunities" they will encounter along the way.

The first two of these strategies were addressed in the previous chapter. We shall deal with the third one here. As before, the evidence in this chapter meets the "moderate-quality" criterion of the GRADE Working Group.*

Scenario

Today's mentoring session opened with the following mentee's lament:

> Yesterday I was brimming with optimism, enthusiasm, and resolve. My morning's emails included the stupendous news that the resubmission of my first-ever RCT grant application has been successful, and I think that one more solid day's effort on the manuscript reporting my first-ever independent systematic review (the one that formed the basis for that successful grant resubmission) can get it ready to send to my favorite journal. And the overseas graduate student I peer-mentored last year reports that, with my help, she has won the scholarship competition that will permit her to finish an advanced degree before she returns home, and the drop-in clinic at the homeless shelter where two colleagues and I volunteer has finally received funding from the city for a nurse-practitioner.

---

* See http://www.gradeworkinggroup.org/.

Mentorship in Academic Medicine, First Edition. Sharon E. Straus and David L. Sackett.
© 2014 John Wiley & Sons, Ltd. Published 2014 by John Wiley & Sons, Ltd.

Finally, I learned that I've just received a teaching award from my junior house staff and medical students.

However, my optimism and resolve took several hits as I scanned the other new emails in my inbox: an automated request (sans abstract) from a journal to review a manuscript they've just received; an invitation from a recently-tenured senior colleague to take over, reorganize, and run his graduate course on adaptive trials; invitations to register for two annual meetings (the Society for Clinical Trials and my sub-specialty society) and two special symposia (in areas of tangential interest), all to be held at attractive destinations; an email request from the dean's executive officer to serve on a committee to re-review and re-reorganize the hospital-university space dispute resolution system; a very generously funded "Request for RCT Proposals" for a disease outside my interests and specialty; a request from a colleague in that specialty to help him apply for those funds; and a plea from a member of my clinical rota to take her call this coming weekend.

At this early "stem cell" point in the mentee's career, they are an omni-potential academic clinician, and their brains, skills, and interests could propel them into a wide array of exciting and fulfilling careers. For example, their experience with the overseas graduate student could inaugurate a career in international health research and education. Or they could evolve into a healthcare innovator and evaluator, attacking problems in personal or public healthcare closer to home. Or, they could evolve into an educational innovator and evaluator, and any of the foregoing could lead to a career in progressively senior administrative and leadership posts.

Regardless of their career path, their professional success and life-satisfaction will depend on their ability to focus their time and energy on their primary professional and social goals. Consequently, they must strictly ration any diversion of their time to the myriad other opportunities that will be offered to or thrust upon them. That is, they will have to learn how to say "no" (nicely) to some opportunities and, especially, to the far more numerous "dys-opportunities" (the tasks that devour their time and energy with little chance of useful results and therefore retard their career and personal development). Helping mentees learn how to do this is a key element of successful mentoring [1].

This process begins with helping mentees address the priority lists described in the previous chapter: Priority Lists #1 (*things you're doing now that you want to quit*) and especially #1a (*things you've just been asked to do that you want to refuse to do*). The key to managing (and helping to manage) these priorities is to identify all those things that mentees really shouldn't do – whether they're already doing them, or whether they've just been asked to do them – and to say "no" to them in a firm but courteous fashion (i.e. nicely).

In that informal survey of about 50 of our colleagues worldwide, we found that not only is this point of view about protecting new academics widely shared, but also identified their strong opinion that established academics (including mentors) retain the need to get better at saying "no" (nicely) to the requests and demands that not only threaten their own continuing careers and satisfaction but also limit their contributions to the careers and satisfaction of others (e.g. limiting ability to take on new mentees).

Because our focus is on the mentoring of mentees, we will stress learning when and how to say "no" early in one's career, and how to say "no" nicely, so as to avoid offending people and other undesirable consequences of saying "no". However, as mentees' careers progress and they become established clinician-scientists and educators (with tenure or its equivalent, with a couple of important papers prominently published, and with enough self-assurance to have achieved the prerequisites for becoming effective mentors themselves) they should contribute and help to support a collaborative scientific and medical culture by saying "yes" to requests for teaching, peer-review, and useful administrative tasks (especially when they benefit younger colleagues).

In this chapter, we tabulate 40 specific dys-opportunities that have befallen us and our colleagues worldwide, as originally described in a "Clinician-trialist round" written by Andrew Oxman and Dave Sackett [1, 2], accompanied by suggestions as to why mentees might benefit from saying "no" to them. They are grouped into conferences, administration, grant applications and other people's research, other people's papers, teaching and supervising, clinical work, working with other people, and reading.

Two points to consider before you go there. First, we offer a trio of caveats for mentees and mentors alike: One, the pursuit of happiness – especially as it results from fulfilling one's sense of professional, social, family, and global responsibilities – will sometimes conflict with one's pursuit of success as an academician. For example, the time and energy devoted to frontline patient care in refugee camps must be subtracted from the time and energy available for designing, executing, and publishing educational and other health research. Both endeavours are worthy, and only the individual assessing them can decide whether and how to apportion their time and energy between them.

In our second caveat, we suggest that every dys-opportunity in the tables has the potential to become a positive experience and significant contribution, not just for others but for oneself, and not just locally but internationally. Accordingly, each table has a third column that suggests when a mentee might want to say "yes" to this potential opportunity. Which leads to our third caveat, directed toward academic clinicians at the start of their careers, when saying "yes" too often delays getting their research launched, conducted, and published, stresses their social and family life, and pushes them toward burn-out. This is where mentors play vital roles in helping them distinguish opportunities from dys-opportunities.

Once mentees have achieved their initial successes, they may want to begin to say "yes" more often. Nonetheless, there are some dys-opportunities that never become worthwhile, and we'll point those out along the way.

Many of the table entries will appear anti-authoritarian or even rebellious, but such attitudes have played important roles in the advance of science [3, 4]. Indeed, Peter Szatmari has written:

> There are certain personal characteristics associated with being a successful clinician-scientist investigator. One must be intensely curious about [the subject], profoundly dissatisfied with the current state of knowledge, and carry a profound desire to know more as a way of helping one's patients. Having personality characteristics associated with *oppositional-defiant disorder*[†] can also be quite helpful [5].

To which Sharon Straus responded with: "This is excellent! And much better to have than the narcissistic personality disorders, which I think many academics have."

Our second point before introducing Tables 4.2.1–4.2.8 is that, to some readers, they may appear unbalanced, pessimistic and cynical. It is not hard to see how it might be perceived in that way. Occasionally saying "yes" to something that is not a priority can turn out to be an unexpected, wonderful experience. To paraphrase Milan Kundera: Was it better to say no or to say yes? "There is no means of testing which decision is better, because there is no basis for comparison [6]." That is what sometimes makes life unbearably light; it is not a randomized trial where you have the opportunity to say both "no" and "yes" and compare the consequences.

However, as a colleague noted: "I have never regretted that I said no to something, but I have often regretted that I said yes." And in the words of Josh Billings: "Half of the troubles of this life can be traced to saying yes too quickly and not saying no soon enough." The problem is that for many the default is to say "yes". We suggest that a mentee's default should be to say "no" and when they say "yes", to say it more slowly.

[†] A pattern of disobedient, hostile, and defiant behavior toward authority figures and requests from adults [read: chairs and deans], best treated by mental health professionals [read: mentors] and family therapy [read: teams].

Table 4.2.1   Conferences (including annual meetings and academic meetings)

What	Why say "no"	Exceptions
Attending a conference	It steals time before, during and afterward, magnifies your carbon footprint and neglect of your family, and rewards you with an over-flowing inbox on your return.	When you have specific goals or opportunities, such as meeting with collaborators or potential collaborators, and those clearly outweigh the lost time, carbon waste, familial neglect, and overflowing inbox.
Speaking at a conference	It takes time to prepare and the benefits rarely outweigh the downsides of attending a conference, if this is your main reason for going.	When you already have a talk that went well elsewhere and other reasons for attending the conference, you have an important message to deliver and the conference provides an outstanding opportunity to deliver that message to an audience that might not otherwise get the message, or you have an opportunity to interact with an important audience.
Chairing a session at a conference	The benefits almost never outweigh the downsides of attending a conference, if this is your main reason for going. If you have other reasons for going, you are stuck going to that session and you are at the mercy of speakers who ramble and run overtime.	When you have other reasons for attending the conference and it is a session that you would want to attend anyway.
Listening to drug-industry-recruited speakers at a nice (holiday) venue (i.e. a boondoggle)	They want to buy (or at least rent) you for the benefit of their stockholders.	Only to repay family members for your past neglect of them.

This chapter would be incomplete if it didn't confront email, that double-edged sword that can both enable and disable academic clinicians at any stage in their mentorships. Many of your most valuable exchanges between mentees and mentors and other colleagues (and most of the requests you've received) probably have occurred via email. And mentees have no

Table 4.2.2 Administration

What	Why say "no"	Exceptions
Administrative and "planning" meetings	They are almost always a waste of your time.	Rarely; when they have clear, worthwhile and achievable goals, you can make an important contribution, and they don't take any more time than what is needed.
Administrative tasks or posts	They steal academic and social time and energy.	When they are part of your contract, they will further your academic or social goals, or they are really interesting and will demonstrate your willingness to "pull your own weight" within your group.
Constantly pointing out problems during staff/ division meetings and sessions with your department head	This can take on a life of its own and waste significant emotional energy. It also does not endear you to your colleagues who also must work under the same conditions.	If, when you approach, you want your boss to think "Here comes trouble!" rather than "Here comes a pissant wuss."*
Holding office in national or international organizations	Can consume too much time and produce too much CO_2.	When you are well-established and can make a contribution that is both unique and consequential.

Adapted by permission of SAGE Publications Ltd., London, Los Angeles, New Delhi, Singapore and Washington DC, from [2] Oxman A, Sackett DL. Clinician-Trialist Rounds 14. Ways to advance your career by saying "no", Part 2: When to say "no," and why. Clinical Trials 2012; 10: 181–87, Copyright ©SAGE Publications Ltd, 2012.
*This exception was submitted by the founding editor of the journal *Clinical Trials*, Curt Meinert.

doubt already appreciated that RCT ideas and preliminary protocols can be exchanged, discussed, and revised with worldwide colleagues within hours, that data-quality checks can be completed swiftly across time zones and work schedules, and that every collaborator who wants to see the latest draft of a research report can get it within seconds.

Moreover, of course, both mentees and mentors are already email beneficiaries in their clinical training and practice, all the more so for those of them who don't automatically receive lab, imaging, and other clinical reports via a hospital information system, or don't have ready access to "experts." For example, "Fast Facts and Concept" emails have been shown to increase US internal medicine interns' knowledge of palliative care topics and self-reported palliative care skills [14]. And a GI trainee in Los Angeles, preparing departmental rounds on confocal laser endomicroscopy, posed

Table 4.2.3 Grant applications and other people's research

What	Why say "no"	Exceptions
Responding to calls for proposals	Responding to calls for proposals that are outside of your primary area of interest takes time away from working on more important projects.	When it is an opportunity to fund a project that you already want to do or sparks a new idea or a new collaboration for a project that you have both the motivation and capacity to do.
Responding to research money offers from industry	You will be serving their stockholders, not your patients or the public, and there is a high risk of losing credibility among your peers and progeny.	When they supplement public funding for your really important research and they cannot revise your protocol, have no access to interim efficacy data and no veto over how you analyze and publish it.[*]
Preparing and submitting a research application with a miniscule chance of success	You could gain at least as much, but waste less time, by betting on horses, football matches, or the Irish lottery.	If you could prepare it in one evening as a "dry run" for a later, serious application for an important project.
Offers to be a co-investigator	You should say no to projects of limited interest to you and to people with little research training (unless they are really brilliant). And, you risk getting labeled by grant reviewers as "involved in too many projects."	When the project is directly relevant to your goals, you'd make an important contribution, you'd enjoy working with these collaborators, you'd learn important new methods, and authorship is specified at the outset.
Consulting on or contributing to trial methods without being a co-investigator or co-author[†]	Most trials require major expert methodologic input, beginning with formulating the question, and suffer in its absence. Consequently this can steal substantial time and energy (or waste it), without giving credit where credit is due.	If it's in your job description or comes with a consultation fee of 'clinical' magnitude.[‡]
Last minute requests to help with a grant application	Ditto. This consumes your free time and there is a higher risk of this being wasted time.	When it's in your job description; give priority to those in your department, and insist that they give you more lead time in the future.
Being a consultant for an ongoing trial or other research project	Much more likely to retard than advance progress toward your primary goals.	When the time required is little and relevance to your goals is large, or the remuneration is of "clinical" magnitude (and you need the money).

Table 4.2.3 (Continued)

What	Why say "no"	Exceptions
Joining your local research ethics committee	This is a time-devourer with the risk of making lethal decisions [7], you might have to work with bullies [8], and it requires tutoring before you take it on.	When your mentor is a member, attend as a silent spectator-learner; later on, join a regional ethics committee that replaces multiple local boards [9], deals with protocols in your area of interest, and is staffed with competent and friendly scientists and ethicists.
Responding to surveys	Most have little scientific merit and they rarely are relevant.	When it is relevant, of high methodological quality, and includes the promise of feedback.
Peer-reviewing grant applications	Why are you taking time away from your own grant applications (especially if you have already reviewed two for every one you've submitted)? A growing problem when departments institute mandatory "internal" grant reviews.	When your mentor also reviews it and you compare notes, it is in your primary areas of expertise and interest, reviewing it will increase your expertise, and you can contribute to improving it (clinicians should document the time spent doing this for CME credits).

Adapted by permission of SAGE Publications Ltd., London, Los Angeles, New Delhi, Singapore and Washington DC, from [2] Oxman A, Sackett DL. Clinician-Trialist Rounds 14. Ways to advance your career by saying "no", Part 2: When to say "no," and why. Clinical Trials 2012; 10: 181–87, Copyright ©SAGE Publications Ltd, 2012.
*But even in these circumstances, they will need to declare this as a competing interest and must be prepared for the perception that they have 'sold out.'
†Biostatisticians and solo trialists in clinical departments are frequently asked to do this.
‡Equivalent to what a specialist physician would bill for spending that time performing clinical consultations.

an academic question about it in one-time emails to 39 US and Canadian experts, received his first answer within 30 minutes, and heard from 77% of them within 13 days [15]. A group of neurologists in Belfast, serving a population of 1.7 million whose average wait for a first neurology appointment was 72 weeks, reduced it to 4 weeks when primary care clinicians emailed their consult requests on a one-page template and quickly received a return email from the consultant with either a diagnosis and management advice, an appointment for investigations, a request for further information (all the former without the patient being seen), or an appointment. They found it safe, changed only three diagnoses on re-referral, and reduced the net cost

Table 4.2.4   Writing, editing, and publishing other people's papers

What	Why say "no"	Exceptions
Peer-reviewing journal manuscripts	Why are you taking time away from your own papers (especially if you have already reviewed two for every one you've submitted)?	When your mentor also reviews it and you compare notes, it is in your primary areas of expertise and interest, reviewing it will increase your expertise, and you can contribute to improving it (clinicians should document the time spent doing this for CME credits).
Offers of co-authorship	Any papers you would not want to read yourself, that you don't think are important, or that you would not want to put your name on are a waste of your time.	When they are of interest to you, you can provide useful input, and you'd enjoy and learn from the other authors.
Writing book chapters	It can take huge amounts of time to properly search for and appraise the literature. Book chapters aren't indexed and are likely to be hard to find. They count little or nothing toward promotion and tenure.	When you've already done most of the work for your thesis, a grant application, or as part of a systematic review.
Editing symposia, special journal issues, or books	This is akin to herding Canada geese in July: participants are noisy (often noisome), hard to organize, often go into hiding, head off in all directions, and leave a terrible mess behind for you to clean up.	When the subject matter is in your primary area of interest, they give you an editorial assistant to do the herding and cleaning up, and you will be named first on the resulting publication.
Media requests for interviews	Journalists often misunderstand, misrepresent, or sensationalize what you say, badger you, press you to meet their deadlines, and may refuse to show you their drafts or make sure they have quoted and interpreted what you said correctly. You will frequently emerge sadder, wiser, and the butt of jokes [1].	When the journalist and media outlet has a good reputation for fact-checking and avoiding hyperbole, or you write and control your own lay presentations, or you have a narcissistic personality disorder.

Table 4.2.5 Teaching and supervising

What	Why say "no"	Exceptions
Organizing a course	The time you'd hoped to spend making the course scientifically and educationally innovative will be almost totally diverted to tracking down and convincing reluctant colleagues to teach and finding meeting rooms not already booked for other purposes.	When your academic career is thriving, the course is at the heart of your academic interests, and you are assigned a seasoned staff assistant with a great track record for getting teachers and room schedulers to make and fulfill commitments.
Being on a thesis committee	This takes time and early in your career may create a conflict of interest with your own ideas and projects.	When your career is well underway, you could uniquely contribute to the student, and there is no conflict of interest, or your university demands it.
Supervising multiple trainee projects	This spreads you so thin that you can't pay enough attention, not only to your own career development, but to each of theirs (when they are even more vulnerable than you are).	When your career is well underway, but never more trainees than you can really serve and still maintain your own progress.
Supervising people, not of your choosing, with (even) less experience than you	People that you didn't choose, with whom you may not be compatible, and who may want to compete with you around your ideas and projects are a time- and energy-sink.	Collaborative people with whom you are compatible, and with whom you would choose to work.
Being the "designated research support person" for a division or department	You risk being totally consumed by the needs of others, with no time and energy for your own academic career, if you are bombarded by requests to assist people (with even less experience than you) with their research.	When your appointment specifies sufficient protected time for your own career, you are able to set up restricted "research support clinic hours" and an appointment system, and your boss pre-agrees to get additional help when your waiting-times hamper your colleagues meeting funding deadlines and running their projects.

Table 4.2.6   Clinical work

What	Why say "no"	Exceptions
Requests from on high to substantially increase your clinical work and billings*	There goes your academic career, your social/family time, or both!	When you desperately need the money and have decided to abandon/curtail either your research career or your social/family time, or when you can't find a better job elsewhere.
Being chief-of-service	Colleagues need to respect (or at least fear) you before they will follow you, and the time you'd hoped to spend improving clinical care and teaching will be largely consumed resolving petty disputes (often unsuccessfully) and dealing with personality disorders.	When improving clinical care and teaching is at the core of your interests and job-description, or when your research career is already well-established.
Requests from colleagues to take over their clinic-session or night call	Saying "yes" requires you to sacrifice either 'protected' research time and productivity, or social/family time.	On compassionate grounds, and in the form of swapping, with payback in full.
Sitting on a clinical guideline panel	Guideline panels may be dominated by members indebted to industry and your reputation may suffer by association, may be poorly chaired or use inappropriate methods, or the guidelines may not be needed.	When the guideline panel is broadly composed [11], the panel does not include conflicted experts, the chair is well-selected and prepared, appropriate methods are used, there are non-industry funds available to support the rigorous methods, the guideline is needed, and you will learn from the experience and be able to contribute.
Seeing a pharmaceutical representative at their request	They are walking drug ads that distort evidence, are often silent about risks, and seek to hook you and your patients on expensive, proprietary drugs.	Virtually none.

Adapted by permission of SAGE Publications Ltd., London, Los Angeles, New Delhi, Singapore and Washington DC, from [2] Oxman A, Sackett DL. Clinician-Trialist Rounds 14. Ways to advance your career by saying "no", Part 2: When to say "no," and why. Clinical Trials 2012; 10: 181–87, Copyright ©SAGE Publications Ltd, 2012.

*The cause for this request needs a diagnosis: Is it the *mentee's* problem (not meeting previously negotiated practice, research, teaching, or administrative targets) or *the institution's* (heading toward bankruptcy)?

Table 4.2.7 Working with other people

What	Why say "no"	Exceptions
Working with disorganized colleagues	They steal time and energy and are likely to fracture friendships.	When you are in control of an important project, they are not damaging the project, and it would take more time and effort to disengage them than to tolerate their disorganization until the project is completed.
Working with famous people who are too busy, too self-involved or too selfish	They are unlikely to teach or mentor you, and might exploit you and steal your ideas.	When it would result in a major career advance, you have a written agreement about authorship before you begin, your mentor is poised to take them on when they mistreat you, and you have a time-limited agreement with an exit strategy.
Working with people you don't like	Why add to life's miseries?	Ditto
Working entirely on your own	Less perspective, less competency in relevant methods, less access to study participants, and less fun.	When you are a super-efficient polymath and you have access to plenty of study participants, have an offensive personality, or you are a misanthrope.
Responding to authority in general	All of the reasons for saying no to different types of requests (in Tables 4.2.1–4.2.6) apply, regardless of who makes the request.*	If you feel unable to say "no" to any of the requests in Tables 4.2.1–4.2.6 simply because it is made by an authority, you should consider looking for a new job or a new mentor.

Adapted by permission of SAGE Publications Ltd., London, Los Angeles, New Delhi, Singapore and Washington DC, from [2] Oxman A, Sackett DL. Clinician-Trialist Rounds 14. Ways to advance your career by saying "no", Part 2: When to say "no," and why. Clinical Trials 2012; 10: 181–87, Copyright ©SAGE Publications Ltd, 2012.
*Some consider an "oppositional defiant disorder" essential to academic success (see text).

per referral by 58% [16]. Finally, the bulk of responses to our survey of our international colleagues for this book were received within 48 hours.

Finally, the numbers and sorts of patients and citizens who are benefitting from the incorporation of email into their care are rapidly rising, from single email delivered, computer-tailored smoking cessation interventions in the Netherlands [17], to email reminders that increase visits for colorectal cancer screening in Oregon [18], to weekly email messages and a monthly personal email message for maintaining weight-loss in England [19], to viral email

Table 4.2.8   Reading

What	Why say "no"	Exceptions
Reading whatever clinical or research literature that comes your way	Most of it* is unreliable or irrelevant [12, 13].	Services that abstract high-quality articles in your field.†
Reading the rest of this chapter or clinical article	Too late! Just as you unlearned what your parents taught you about having to finish eating everything on your dinner plate, you need to unlearn having to finish reading every chapter or article just because you started it.	Only if you are trying to avoid other tasks but want to appear deep in thought.

Adapted by permission of SAGE Publications Ltd., London, Los Angeles, New Delhi, Singapore and Washington DC, from [2] Oxman A, Sackett DL. Clinician-Trialist Rounds 14. Ways to advance your career by saying "no", Part 2: When to say "no," and why. Clinical Trials 2012; 10: 181–87, Copyright ©SAGE Publications Ltd, 2012.
*"Generally, a clinical reader would need to read in the range of 13–14 articles from [the] top 20 journals to obtain one that is directly clinically important in any health care area, although the range is substantial (1.1 to 36.9). We call this number the "number of articles needed to be read" or NNR."[13]
†We both subscribe to EvidenceUpdates: http://plus.mcmaster.ca/EvidenceUpdates /AboutThisSite.aspx.

marketing as a distribution method for tobacco control advertisements in Australia [10].

But this last example exposes email's second edge, exemplified by the Maltese hospital-based pediatrician who monitored a month of personal emails (back in 2008) and concluded that 70% were spam [21]. Was Albert Einstein anticipating email as far back as 1917 when he wrote to a friend "Our much-praised technological progress ... could be compared to an axe in the hand of a pathological criminal."?[22] We suspect most of you have held a similar thought as you faced an ever-bloated email inbox whose uninvited, unwelcome contents – if thoroughly answered – would devour your time, exhaust your energy, and extinguish your fun day after day after day.

What solutions are there for saying "no" (nicely) to unsolicited email? We close this chapter with some generic strategies and tactics we and our colleagues employ and recommend to our mentees [2].

• Never work for a boss (including yourself!) who declares that you are "unprofessional" if you don't respond to all email within a day.

- Initiate – and keep up to date – personal email countermeasures that ban the same unsolicited email from ever appearing a second – or certainly a third – time in your inbox. These strategies range from hitting "unsubscribe" options at the first opportunity, to using your mail user agent (Microsoft, Mozilla, or whatever) options to ban further messages from a source that bothers you twice, to employing ever more elaborate spam-detectors (rumor has it the Bayesian ones are best at killing guilty messages while sparing the innocent ones [23]).

- Try to "touch" every inbox message just once by either: replying to it with a short answer; highlighting and filing it in a dated "To do" file for a long answer; filing it in an archive for future reference; deleting it, or deleting it and banning its repetition. The secondary objective here is experiencing the exhilaration that comes from seeing an empty inbox.

- Employ, depending on the severity of your email affliction, progressively restrictive auto-replies based on the "I'm away at a meeting or on vacation"‡ model (but avoiding the fatal flaw of accumulating a mountain of email waiting to paralyze the returning attendee or vacationer). These auto-replies can range all the way from: "I am unable to respond to email for the next x days/weeks. If your inquiry is still timely after that date, please write to me again at that time" to "I am unable to respond to current email messages."§ Of course, you still read your email (thus avoiding the fatal flaw), touching each one once, responding to just the ones you find important and deleting all the rest.

How to say "No" (nicely)

Again drawing on previous work [24], we close this chapter with some tactics that mentees can be taught for saying "no" nicely. And, once again, we confront the possibility that this advice may come across as selfish and cynical to some readers. From our perspective, the issue is not that some wonderful and worthy opportunities and experiences can be lost by saying "no" when they are offered to mentees; of course they can. The issue is that, by

---

‡ Note that this out of office email can be used not just for vacations but for when you're on clinical service and you know that you're going to be swamped and unable to keep up with your inbox.

§ The colleague who suggested this extreme auto-response wrote: "It really works... I just wish I had the fortitude to use it more often. But when I do, it works soooooooo well."

saying "yes" too often, mentees run the risk of over-commitment, over-work, under-achievement across the board, under-socialization, under-enjoyment, failure to deliver on their commitments, and burnout.

Even a superficial literature scan confirms the burnout epidemic. A recent survey of academic internists at the Mayo Clinic (with a response rate indicating that less than a fifth of them had learned how to say "no" to completing questionnaires) found that 30% felt "burned out from my work" at least once a week [25]. The strongest predictors of their burnout were the number of working hours per week, work/home conflicts, and resolving work/home conflicts in favor of work (indicating that their families were paying a price as well). A major cause of burnout was saying "yes" to tasks outside their areas of primary interest, and their risk of burnout doubled when the time available for their highest academic priority shrank to less than 20% of their week [26]. Burnout is even affecting a disturbing proportion of academic clinicians while they are still trainees, postdocs, going for degrees, and in early career development programs. In the degree-granting and career development program at the Clinical and Translational Science Institute of the University of Pittsburgh School of Medicine, 24% of medical students, 12% of residents, 18% of fellows, and 23% of faculty were already experiencing burnout symptoms that wouldn't go away, or felt completely burned out and wondered if they could go on. Work/family imbalances were a frequent cause, especially among women [27].

At one extreme, a recent article describing a faculty survey at 26 US medical schools bore the alarmist title: "Why are a quarter of faculty considering leaving academic medicine?"[28] At the other extreme, the rate of severe burnout among medical school deans, who have survived early burnout and who have become supremely adept at avoiding dys-opportunities by getting others to say "yes" to taking most of them over, was only 2% [29].

Accordingly, until the pursuit of clinical, educational and research excellence, self-efficacy, work-life-family balance, and fun are delisted from the bill of rights of academic clinicians – and until deans, chairs and service chiefs consistently provide sufficient resources to take on additional tasks (however enticing they may be) – mentors will continue to counsel mentees to say "no" (nicely) to most invitations to take on unsolicited assignments.

The advice offered here is a distillate of what colleagues around the world told Andy Oxman and Dave Sackett they said (or wish they'd said instead of accepting what turned out to be major dys-opportunities). As with other chronic maladies, our suggested approach to responding to dys-opportunities involves "stepped care" (Box 4.2.1).

Box 4.2.1 Stepped care for responding to dys-opportunities

Step 1 Don't say "yes" right away.
Step 2 Don't let yourself be flattered or badgered into saying "yes."
Step 3 Make sure you know what is expected.
Step 4 Consider the opportunity cost.
Step 5 Say "no" nicely.
Step 6 Learn from your mistakes.

Adapted by permission of SAGE Publications Ltd., London, Los Angeles, New Delhi, Singapore and Washington DC, from [24] Oxman A, Sackett DL. Clinician-Trialist Rounds: 15. Ways to advance your career by saying "no". Part 3: How to say "no," nicely. *Clinical Trials* 2013, **10** (2) 340–343, Copyright ©SAGE Publications Ltd, 2013.

Step 1 is to advise mentees to resist the temptation to say "yes" immediately to a request, even if it's for something they'd like to do. If they already know that they shouldn't or don't want to do it, they can go to Step 5.

Step 2 is not to let flattery or badgering get the requester anywhere. Mentees can silence it with the simple statement: "If you need my answer right away, it has to be 'no.'" If the badgering continues, mentees can go to Step 5.

Step 3 is for mentees to make sure that they can make a well-informed decision. If they think they might want to say "yes" to a request, they should immediately make a counter-request for written details about precisely what they are being asked to do, with what final product, by what deadline, and with what resources. If mentees don't get sufficient information from this counter-request, they should go to Step 5.

Step 4 is to make sure saying "yes" to a request is worth the opportunity cost. If mentees are not confident it is, they should go to Step 5. But if they think it might be worth the opportunity cost, they should be advised to haul out (and update if necessary) their periodic priority lists from the previous chapter, determine what they'll have to sacrifice from Lists #2 (things they're not doing that they want to start doing) or #3 (things they're doing that they want to continue doing) to take on this new opportunity, and – if so – whether it's worth it. If it isn't, they should go to Step 5.

Mentors (and families[||]) can play a major role in helping mentees make these decisions, and mentors can be vital in backing them up. Mentors can

---

[||] By 'family' we mean the people – closely linked to the mentee through genetics, companionship, or deep friendship – with whom they share vital, mutually nurturing relationships.

help mentees sharpen their assessment of the pros and cons of the "possible pro-opportunity." They can also help mentees distinguish the frisson of "wanting to be wanted" to take on a prestigious dys-opportunity from the sober realization of their sacrifice some family responsibilities, time, talent, energy, fun, and peace-of-mind in order to take it on.

Step 5 is to say "no" nicely. If appropriate, the sting of a mentee's rejection can be tempered by acknowledging the importance of the request, employing phrases like those in Box 4.2.2.

Box 4.2.2 Ways of tempering a rejection

- I'm flattered to be asked but, unfortunately…
- It's very generous of you to offer to include me, but…
- Your work (request) sounds interesting and important, but…
- I know this is important for you, but…

Adapted by permission of SAGE Publications Ltd., London, Los Angeles, New Delhi, Singapore and Washington DC, from [24] Oxman A, Sackett DL. Clinician-Trialist Rounds: 15. Ways to advance your career by saying "no". Part 3: How to say "no," nicely. *Clinical Trials* 2013, **10** (2) 340–343, Copyright ©SAGE Publications Ltd, 2013.

Box 4.2.3 lists the verbatim responses our colleagues and we use when we say "no." They can be used to complete the sentences in Box 4.2.2, or on their own. As mentees can see, there are so many highly appropriate reasons why their other responsibilities make it impossible to take on dys-opportunities, that they don't need to make one up. Phoney excuses, once exposed, will damage your mentee's credibility and reputation. As well, they are tougher to remember than true ones, as pointed out by "Honest Abe" Lincoln: [††] "No man has a good enough memory to make a successful liar."[3]

If possible, mentees should also provide constructive advice. Their best advice would be to identify other individuals or groups who could help. But they should be careful never to "throw any friends under the bus" by nominating them to a lousy dys-opportunity being controlled by a frowsy tyrant. And, it's both collegial and helpful to "cc" or "bcc" your nominee on the email response so that they are forewarned about a possible request.

[††] An attitude of mind converted to a virtue by Mark Twain: "I am different from [George] Washington; I have a higher, grander standard of principle. Washington could not lie. I can lie, but I won't." [http://www.quoteidea.com/authors/mark-twain-quotes]

Box 4.2.3 Ways of saying "no" nicely (verbatim)

1 Just say "no":
- I can't.
2 I simply don't have enough time:
- I'm too busy.
- My plate is full.
- I'm not available due to prior commitments.
- Prior commitments prevent me from making a meaningful contribution.
- I am swamped right now. Best of luck.
- In light of all my other commitments I can't give this the attention it deserves.
- I can't in good conscience take this on since I am already over committed.
- The timing just doesn't work for me.
- You should have come to me sooner (for last-minute requests). I don't have time to do this now.
- I really want to do this, but I've said yes to too many things (or I have hit a pre-specified limit) and it has gotten me into trouble (or I will compromise a prior commitment).
3 I'm not allowed:
- My mentor (or boss) won't let me.
- My mentor has me working on a ton of stuff such that I don't see my partner and kids.
- I have already [e.g. supervised two students] this year, which is the quota set by my mentor (boss).
4 I need to focus elsewhere:
- At this point in my career I need to focus on my research.
- I can't take this [e.g. teaching] on now. It is something I would like to do and plan on doing more of when my research is off the ground.
- This was agreed ahead of time and I am being paid less as a researcher [In response to requests to take on additional clinical work that cuts into your mentee's protected research time].
5 It wouldn't be fair to others:
- I already have several students and taking on another would spread me so thinly that it would not help the new student in the way intended and would diminish my ability to help the others.
- I cannot take any more time away from my patients (if I do this the quality of patient care will suffer).
- I can only do this if I can find some mechanism of being relieved of my current administrative responsibilities.
6 It's simply not worth it:
- e.g. based on the abstract, the paper (or grant application) is not worth refereeing.
7 I'm the wrong person to ask:
- I have a conflict of interest.
- I am already working on something similar with another group of colleagues and it would be unfair on them to [do what you have asked].

8 I've nothing to contribute:
  • I would love to contribute to this constructively, but there are so many good people involved I could not possibly add anything.
  • It looks like you have got this taped and I would have very little to add.
  • I don't have the skills or expertise to do what you are asking.
9 Get back to me later:
  • I'd be happy to help, if you get back to me when you've [done whatever the requester should have done and may be unlikely ever to do].
  • Sorry, I don't schedule more than 6 (or 5, or 4 . . .) months in advance lest other unbreakable commitments come up that might force me to renege on this wonderful offer. Please get back to me then.
  • I'd be happy to, what would you like me to give up in its place? [If their boss is asking them to do more than they can manage].

Adapted by permission of SAGE Publications Ltd., London, Los Angeles, New Delhi, Singapore and Washington DC, from [24] Oxman A, Sackett DL. Clinician-Trialist Rounds: 15. Ways to advance your career by saying "no". Part 3: How to say "no," nicely. *Clinical Trials* 2013, **10** (2) 340–343, Copyright ©SAGE Publications Ltd, 2013.

Step 6 is to help mentees learn from their mistakes. If, by ignoring or mis-applying the foregoing, they find themselves sacrificing work and family time, creative energy, and fun as they slog through a dys-opportunity, they should be advised to get to work on extricating themselves via Priority List #4 (Strategies for improving the balance within their lists by shortening Lists #1 and #1a (*quit* and *refuse*) over the next 6 months), and – once (more) bitten – vow to be twice shy next time.

Bottom line and scenario resolution

Your mentee said "no" nicely to this array of dys-opportunities in the following ways:
• *The automated request (sans abstract) from a journal to review a manuscript they've just received*: Raised at the conclusion of a regular mentoring session, she acknowledged that she'd already refereed three papers this year, that the journal was not one in which she'd want to publish her own work, and that they failed to provide enough information for her to determine whether she'd have anything to offer as a reviewer. On the bus home, she pulled up the request on her iPhone, ticked the "refuse" box, and deleted the original request. Time required: minutes.
• *The invitation from a recently-tenured senior colleague to take over, reorganize, and run his graduate course on adaptive trials*: She discusses this with you in person at a mentoring session. She respects this person, and would enjoy running this course later in her career (but not now), and doesn't want to offend him. You agree with her assessment and together you sort out a counter-proposal: she declines the full offer (citing you as advising against

it, to make it clear than she'd taken senior advice and that he'd have to deal with you if he tried to pressure her), but offers to give one session toward the end of the course. Time required to discuss and respond: 2 hours, including sending you a draft of her counter-proposal, spread over a week.

- *The invitations to register for two annual meetings (the Society for Clinical Trials and my sub-specialty society) and two special symposia (in areas of tangential interest), all to be held at attractive destinations*: Brought up and quickly disposed at a regular mentoring session, she has attended the first two previously and acknowledges little marginal gain from further passive attendance. However, she's already prepared abstracts for the first two and the meetings will provide the opportunity to meet with some collaborators who live in that country. She decides to attend them if her abstracts are selected for oral presentations (and will bring along other protocols and manuscripts to work on during flights and between sessions). She'll pass on the latter two meetings. Time required: minutes.

- *The email request from the Dean's exec officer to serve on a committee to re-review and re-reorganize the hospital–university space-dispute resolution system*: Handled in seconds by the two of you agreeing that this is a total waste of her time. She emails the exec officer that, after reviewing her current contributions and obligations, you have prohibited her from taking on this task. Time required: minutes.

- *The very generously funded "Request for RCT Proposals" for a disease outside my specialty*: She instantly realizes that although she could draft a protocol in one day, she'd have to spend several more assembling CVs, letters of support, budgets, signatures, and the like. Tacking this on to her regular agenda item about her current research progress, she decides she already has enough grant support to spend all her available research time for the next 2+ years in exciting and fruitful ways, and decides not to apply. Time required: minutes.

- *The request from a colleague in that specialty to help him apply for those funds*: Adding this to the agenda of a regular mentoring session, she describes wanting to help a friend but expresses doubts about this person's research competency and fears that she might get sucked into doing the heavy lifting on the grant and carrying the majority of the responsibility for conducting the study. After discussion, she decides to email her colleague, asking him to send her his first complete draft within the next month (one month ahead of the grant deadline) and, if and when she receives it, promises to give him a "one-off" set of comments and suggestions, but declines to be a co-applicant or co-investigator. Time required: Minutes to discuss and write the email, and she never receives a draft protocol.

- *The "tweety" plea from a member of my clinical rota to take her call this coming weekend*: Following a 20-second discussion as she was leaving your meeting, and because she had no plans for this weekend, she texts her provisional agreement to the plea while waiting for the elevator, but stipulates that it won't be activated until her colleague texts her back, agreeing to pay back in full by taking your mentee's call the next weekend. Tweety reply time required: 20 seconds.

References

1. Oxman A, Sackett DL. Clinician-trialist rounds: 13. Ways to advance your career by saying "no" Part 1: Why to say "no" (nicely), and saying "no" to email. Clin Trials J 2012; 9: 806–8.
2. Oxman A, Sackett DL. Clinician-trialist rounds: 14. Ways to advance your career by saying "no", Part 2: When to say "no," and why. Clin Trials J 2012; 10: 181–87.
3. Chalmers I. Scientific inquiry and authoritarianism in perinatal care and education. Birth 1983; 10: 151–62.
4. Oxman AD, Guyatt GH. The science of reviewing research. Ann NY Acad Sci 1993; 703: 125–34.
5. Szatmari P. Personal communication. Sept 2012.
6. Kundera M. *The Unbearable Lightness of Being*. New York: Harper & Row, 1984.
7. Roberts I, Prieto-Merino D, Shakur H, *et al*. Effect of consent rituals on mortality in emergency care research. Lancet 2011; 377: 1071–2.
8. Sokol DK. Is bioethics a bully? BMJ 2012; 345: 32.
9. Ontario Cancer Research Ethics Board website. Available at: http://oicr.on.ca/oicr-programs-and-platforms/ontario-cancer-research-ethics-board. Accessed 30 Sept 2012.
10. Sackett D, Guyatt G, Haynes B, Tugwell P. Dealing with the media. In: Haynes RB, Sackett DL, Guyatt GH, Tugwell P. *Clinical Epidemiology: How to Do Clinical Practice Research*, 3rd edn. Philadelphia: Lippincott Williams & Wilkins, 2006; pp 474–86.
11. Fretheim A, Schünemann HJ, Oxman AD. Improving the use of research evidence in guideline development: 3. Group composition. Health Res Policy Syst 2006; 4: 15.
12. McKibbon KA, Wilczynski NL, Haynes RB. What do evidence-based secondary journals tell us about the publication of clinically important articles in primary health care journals? BMC Medicine 2004, 2: 33.
13. Purpose and procedure. Evid Based Med 2012;17:e4 doi:10.1136/ebmed.17.01.e4.
14. Claxton R, Marks S, Buranosky R, *et al*. The educational impact of weekly e-mailed fast facts and concepts. J Palliat Med 2011; 14: 475–81.
15. Paul N. Use of email to acquire information from experts. Lancet 2011; 377: 208.
16. Patterson V, Humphreys J, Henderson M, Crealey G. Email triage is an effective, efficient and safe way of managing new referrals to a neurologist. Qual Saf Health Care 2010; 19: e51.
17. Te Poel F, Bolman C, Reubsaet A, de Vries H. Efficacy of a single computer-tailored e-mail for smoking cessation: results after 6 months. Health Educ Res. 2009; 24: 930–40.
18. Muller D, Logan J, Dorr D, Mosen D. The effectiveness of a secure email reminder system for colorectal cancer screening. AMIA Annu Symp Proc 2009: 457–61.
19. Thomas D, Vydelingum V, Lawrence J. E-mail contact as an effective strategy in the maintenance of weight loss in adults. J Hum Nutr Diet. 2011; 24: 32–8.

20. Carter OB, Donovan R, Jalleh G. Using viral e-mails to distribute tobacco control advertisements: an experimental investigation. J Health Commun. 2011; 16: 698–707.

21. Grech V, Hugo AM. Email spam: a single user's perspective. J Vis Comm Med 2008; 31: 110–2.

22. Lightman A. *A Sense of the Mysterious: Science and the Human Spirit.* New York: Pantheon, 2005; p. 110.

23. Wikipedia contributors. Bayesian spam filtering. Wikipedia, The Free Encyclopedia. July 12, 2012, 16:00 UTC. Available at: http://en.wikipedia.org/w/index .php?title=Bayesian_spam_filtering&oldid=501901515. Accessed October 15, 2012.

24. Oxman A, Sackett DL. Clinician-trialist rounds: 15. Ways to advance your career by saying "no". Part 3: How to say "no," nicely. Clinical Trials J 2013, 10: 340–43.

25. Dyrbye LN, West CP, Satele D, *et al.* Work/home conflict and burnout among academic internal medicine physicians. Arch Intern Med 2011; 171: 1207–9.

26. Tait D, Shanafelt TD, Boone S, *et al.* Burnout among academic faculty. Arch Intern Med 2012; 172: 1377–85.

27. Primack BA, Dilmore TC, Switzer GE, *et al.* Burnout among early career clinical investigators. Clin Transl Sci. 2010; 3: 186–8.

28. Pololi LH, Krupat E, Civian JT, *et al.* Why are a quarter of faculty considering leaving academic medicine? A study of their perceptions of institutional culture and intentions to leave at 26 representative U.S. medical schools. Acad Med 2012; 87: 859–69.

29. Gabbe SG, Webb LE, Moore DE, *et al.* Burnout in medical school deans: an uncommon problem. Acad Med 2008; 83: 476–82.

30. Quotation Collection website. Abraham Lincoln quotes. Available at: http:// www.quotationcollection.com/author/Abraham_Lincoln/quotes. Accessed 18 November 2012.

Chapter 4.3 **Some effective mentoring strategies and tactics**

Part 3: Mentoring for knowledge generation

Scenario

Your peaceful writing day is interrupted by a distressed and distressing telephone call from a very promising mentee, who reports that their first-ever grant application has been turned down. They are devastated (it's their first setback in a promising career), distraught, and wonder if they have chosen the wrong profession. What can and should you do to mentor them through this crisis?

The cardinal measure of a clinical researcher's stature, reputation, and academic success is their generation of new knowledge that carries immediate or eventual benefit to human health. Accordingly, the cardinal measure of the success of these individual's mentors is their ability to nurture and prepare academic clinicians for achieving this success, including mentoring them through the agonies and ecstasies of winning grant support for their research. This chapter, written mostly for mentors of clinician-scientists, will address the lows as well as the highs of winning that support.

Effective mentors begin by displaying and communicating their own enjoyment and love of scientific exploration. They also seize opportunities to introduce their mentees to charismatic leaders performing leading-edge research in their clinical field. Effective mentees catch this "infectious enthusiasm" and start mining their clinical encounters, rounds, seminars, readings, and private musings for questions that need answers:

- Is this "classic" physical finding of tracheal descent really reproducible in patients like mine, and does it accurately rule in or rule out chronic airflow limitation? [1]
- Does this change in a six-minute walk in heart failure patients like mine really indicate a major worsening of their prognosis?

Mentorship in Academic Medicine, First Edition. Sharon E. Straus and David L. Sackett.
© 2014 John Wiley & Sons, Ltd. Published 2014 by John Wiley & Sons, Ltd.

- Does this new anti-thrombotic drug regimen really reduce both bleeds and recurrences following deep vein thrombosis?
- Might my persistently-symptomatic COPD patient who is now taking four meds really feel and function better on just three of them? [2]
- How long does it take stroke patients like mine to actually receive thrombolytics at my hospital?
- Could "motion magnification" replace surface and invasive monitors during obstetrical labor and in neonatal and adult ICUs?
- Is there a better way of teaching patient-centered decision-making to my clinical clerks and evaluating whether they've mastered it?
- Do my palliative care patients experience different responses from their care-givers to requests for analgesics than for anxiolytics?
- In what circumstances does a school feeding program targeting elementary school age children enhance education and health outcomes?
- Does implementation of an evidence-based early mobilization strategy for older adults admitted to acute care hospitals decrease length of stay, increase functional status, and decrease admission to long-term care?
- How can interprofessional education be optimized for undergraduate medical education?
- Does a rapid assessment clinic for patients referred from the Emergency Department with acute exacerbations of chronic diseases lead to decreased admission to hospital and improved quality of care?

Placed on the agendas of mentorship meetings, these primordial ideas can be brought there and explored in three dimensions. First, they can be subjected to the "so what?" test. Would answering the question really make a significant difference to clinical and health care? If so, the second dimension explores whether current methods and resources could be assembled to answer it. And, if so, a search of the current literature and RCT and systematic review registries (like *ClinicalTrials.gov* and PROSPERO) could follow to supply the third dimension of the current state of knowledge and whether the question has already been, or is being, answered.

As a result, effective mentees generate and maintain a ranked list of significant, answerable research questions. Some can be answered by conducting systematic reviews of the pre-existing literature. Others might be answerable through N-of-1 trials. Most, however, will require forming a team, generating a formal protocol, and applying for external funding.

The authors of this book believe that generating, submitting, and defending a research grant is so fundamental a process in the education of an academic clinician scientist that its initial effort should occur as part of their graduate training, and not wait until they are scrambling to get research going as a new postdoc or faculty member. It is highly challenging and time-consuming to prepare a grant application, and just getting to know how the online grant application process works is an important goal for any graduate student or fellow.

Although most funding agencies don't allow graduate students or fellows to be principal applicants on grants, they can appear as paid staff and, by prior agreement, become the lead authors in the presentations and publications generated from the research.*

At the same time that mentees are generating their research agendas, effective mentors provide or arrange for them to receive practical research experience on a productive and congenial research team, where they can learn about how to form and lead their own teams. The mentee's observations about the structure, financing, administration (including hiring and firing of personnel), documentation, and behavior of the various team members (including delegation, credit-sharing, and conflict-resolution) become topics for discussion at mentorship meetings.

Effective mentors who carry out ethical and scientific reviews of outside grants provide opportunities for their mentees to carry out their own duplicate "blind" reviews for later comparison and discussion. This experience can not only sharpen mentees' scientific acumen but also help them develop their own rigorous but civilized and constructive styles of generating useful feedback for use in their later careers.

When compelling and exciting research questions both pass the "so what?" test and are within the mentee's competency to answer, effective mentors play a vital role in helping mentees over their toughest, most demanding, and most important hurdle: generating an unambiguous, answerable research question. Because the words in the research question determine not only the strategy and tactics of the study methods, but also the analysis, interpretation, and credibility of the study results, they deserve days if not weeks of discussion, challenge, and revision at mentorship meetings.

Mentors can help their mentees recognize that the form of their study question varies with the intent of their study. For example, questions about the comparative efficacy or effectiveness of interventions benefit from the PICOT format:

---

* A note of caution here – we've seen many cases where postdoctoral fellows have written grants for their supervisor without receiving authorship or other credit, and we insist that our mentees have discussions with their supervisors about intellectual properties arising from the grant, ensure that they stay involved with the project after their fellowship has been completed, and receive written guarantees about authorship. The best option is for the PI/supervisor (remaining as the Co-PI) to sign the grant over to the postdoctoral fellow once they have an academic job.

P = Patients: Among this specific sort of patient (diagnosis, stage, symptoms, signs, lab data, prognostic factors, etc.) Note that this could also be used to indicate a group or population (such as school-age children, policy makers, clinicians, health care regions etc.)

I = Intervention: Does this specific intervention (drug, device, operation, teaching, talking, etc.)

C = Comparison: Compared to this specific alternative intervention (including an "attention placebo" or nothing at all)

O = Outcome: Improve this specific outcome (survival, clinical event, level of function, quality of life, quality of care, cost etc.)

T = Time: Over this specific period of time?

This same approach can be used for qualitative research questions:

P = Among these patients/providers/policy-makers/participants, population, problem, policy intentions or uses, program

I = Do these health services interventions

C = Under these circumstances, context, concept

O = Affect these barriers, facilitators, attitudes, beliefs, knowledge

Once a mentee has generated a coherent, answerable question, effective mentors guide them through the process of generating a grant application (enlisting critiques and advice from other methodologists, project managers, and budget officers along the way) and shepherd them through all the research ethics committees, institutional review boards, and over the myriad other bureaucratic hurdles. Mentors also see to it that repeated, rigorous critiques of mentees' draft grants are carried out, both by them and by their expert peers.

Several resources are available that describe and proscribe the contents, strategies, and tactics of writing research grants, and their requirements vary so widely between granting bodies that we will not describe them here, other than to point out that some agencies, such as the United States National Institutes of Health, provide a wide array of guides and tips for writing grant applications [3]. Many funding agencies host grant-writing workshops, and trainees should take advantage of these. Effective mentors also share examples of successful grants with their mentees; if mentors are reluctant to share intellectual property with others not involved with the grant, this becomes a perfect opportunity to discuss intellectual property, confidentiality agreements, and the like.

We hold strong opinions about the growing trend for research-intensive departments and institutions to offer "grant-writing" services to their members. On the one hand, these services can helpfully generate those crucial (but mind-numbing) bits of grants that satisfy the ranks of institutional mandarins and lawyers, without whose approval a grant will never see the light of day. On the other hand, they should never be relied upon to generate the study question or protocol – that is not only the mentee's responsibility, but also their unique contribution, and the source of their education. Indeed, we believe one of the unique and most enjoyable aspects of being an academic researcher is the ability to ask and answer questions, and we regard the offloading of this activity to a grant-writing service is an abdication of one's responsibility as a principal investigator. So, offloading the seemingly endless "fussy" bits preparing appendices, tracking down letters of support etc. are fine, but we maintain that forming the study question and laying down the scientific strategies and tactics for answering it are not only the most enjoyable tasks, but ones that should never be handed over to a service bureau.

Another reason to recommend writing a first grant as a graduate student is to confront mentees with how long it takes to move it through their institution's peer review, administrative, and signature processes. The latter two can take two to three weeks to obtain, and internal peer review over a month, so that a grant due September 1st better be ready to submit locally by the 1st of July.

Finally, a key element of good mentoring around a new grant application educates and insulates the mentee (the latter as much as one can) about not only the likelihood of rejection on the first round but also the far brighter prospects on the second. To be sure, a defining moment in any research-stream mentee's career is winning approval of their first research grant application. Not only does it provide them with resources for executing their protocol and generating new knowledge, it also confirms – not only to them but to their colleagues, their institution, and their profession – that they are competent scientists worthy of respect and attention.

However, winning any grant competition is a struggle, and initial applications from even seasoned, successful investigators routinely get turned down. Although there are myriad instructional sources – often from granting agencies themselves – to demonstrate and aid mentees in preparing their research grant applications, there are very few to help them resurrect one that has been rejected, and almost none to help them cope with the psychological trauma of receiving a rejection notice. Because the mentor's role is central, not only to rehabilitating the rejected mentee, but also to resurrecting their rejected application, this chapter will address both of these challenges.

A reprise of the opening scenario

Your peaceful writing day is interrupted by a distressed and distressing tele-phone call from a very promising mentee, who reports that their first-ever grant application has been turned down. They are devastated (it's their first setback in a promising career), distraught, and wonder if they have chosen the wrong profession. What can and should you do to mentor them through this crisis?

Seasoned (scarred?) mentors will have "inoculated" their mentees, well before their applications were submitted, with not only their risks of rejection but the reassurance that similar fates befall initial applications submitted by even highly successful senior investigators. This inoculation can soften, but never eliminate, the blow to the mentee. Accordingly, the rest of this chapter will describe the strategies and tactics that mentors can employ in helping their mentees deal with both the emotional and practical consequences of having their grant application rejected. Although the example we'll use is an application for a randomized trial, the issues and recommendations apply equally to other research designs.

First, mentors can help their mentees recognize (as normal) and deal with the stages of their emotional responses to grant rejection [4]:

1 Their first stage will be dominated by an overwhelming sense of disappointment. It feels like a personal judgment on their scientific abilities, but this can often extend to feeling it is a judgment on their character and personality. Mentors can help mentees by labeling these feelings as normal and even healthy. This reassurance can be accompanied by a strong encouragement to avoid making any important decisions in the first few hours or days after receiving that rejection letter, during which their mentee's ability to critically assess the situation is likely to be clouded. Mentees can be encouraged to shorten the duration of this stage by moving the rejection notice to a folder where it won't glare at them, to turn to their support system of family and friends, and to spend a bit of time in social or athletic pursuits.

2 Their second stage will be dominated by anger, during which they typically "review" the reviewers. How could the reviewers be so stupid! The buggers obviously know nothing! Their comments are so unfair. Did they grasp the originality or the importance of the proposal? Did they *really* understand the objectives and methods? Were they familiar enough with the field or the methodology? Have they truly provided a scientifically accurate review? The answer to at least one of these questions is almost invariably

"no", and provides enough fuel to be angry at the reviewer and the granting agency for some time to come. Some mentees may find that writing a response at this stage (but then putting it away, out of sight) can be helpful, both to dissipate their anger and to provide a starting point for a later, more considered, response. Others may prefer continuing to spend time with their support system and in non-academic activities.

3 Their third stage will be devoted to attempting to reconcile the objectives and methods they presented in their application with the criticisms it received from its reviewers. Although occasional flashbacks to earlier stages may occur, most mentees will become able to respond rationally to the situation they now face.

Next, mentors can help their mentees start this process by encouraging them, first of all, to decide whether their grant application ought to be resurrected. Of course, the chances of getting their grant funded are now better since they know what the reviewers of the agency are thinking. But do they really have a chance to get them to turn their thinking around? The grounds for abandoning the proposal are four:

1 Is the study they proposed *too late*? Did their rejection provide convincing evidence that somebody else has beaten your mentee to the punch and already answered their question? If so, should they abandon this application (for, say, an explanatory trial) and turn their thinking to developing one that addresses the next logical question about the benefits of this experimental treatment (say, by proposing a pragmatic trial)?

2 Is the study they proposed *too early*? Did their rejection provide compelling evidence that your mentee's proposed intervention is too little understood to be ready for testing with their proposed research design? Again, if so, should they abandon this application and develop one (perhaps with a basic scientist co-investigator) that would fill in these blanks?

3 Did their grant receive a ghastly rating for a *fatal flaw* that they simply cannot fix? For example, did the only agency that supports trials like theirs express a crushing lack of interest in their proposal?

4 Would it take *too much of their time* away from worthier pursuits to fix this grant? Has this research project lost its scientific value and attractiveness to your mentee in the interim, replaced by a more important and exciting research question that would be far more deserving of their time and effort?

But if the study they proposed wasn't too late, too early, too uninteresting, or too time-consuming to fix, it's time to help your mentee convert their distress at its rejection into positive efforts to resurrect and resubmit it. In the following paragraphs, we will summarize the strategies and tactics used by over 50 researchers and mentees as they repair and resubmit their unsuccessful research grant proposals [5].

The resurrection process occurs in four stages. Along the way, mentees can be encouraged to take comfort in the fact that many seasoned investigators consider getting a research grant a two-stage process, with stage one ending in a rejected first application.[†]

Stage I. Steps to take *before* mentees meet with colleagues who can help them

A Mentees should alert their co-applicants, mentor, and anybody else they want to involve in their revision and reapplication team (the "R&R team"), and schedule an urgent meeting with them.[‡] In the meanwhile, mentees should do the following homework:

B Mentees should get as much feedback as possible from the granting agency. So that they gain both experience and confidence, mentees should ask for help from their mentors only if absolutely necessary.

   1 Is this the mentee's second or greater rejection of this same grant? If they've passed the "rejection of no return" policy of that agency, it's time to move to another agency or another idea.

   2 If the agency appoints staff "minders" or scientific officers to keep track of individual applications as they go through the review process, mentees can speak with theirs and make thorough notes on what they learn about what went wrong. If the scientific officers created notes on the review, a copy of those notes should be requested (since it may contain vital information not included in the external and internal reviews).

   3 Mentees can find out whether their grant ever got to a peer-review committee, or whether it was rejected before it got there. In the latter case, mentees can try to find out why; one of the author's senior colleagues suggests politely asking them to at least send it for external review, providing a list of knowledgeable reviewers.

   4 Mentees can find out which committee reviewed it and, if possible, the names (or at least the disciplines) of its members. Was it the most appropriate one, or should you request a different review committee when you resubmit?

[†] We think the record is probably held by an antipodean researcher whose application for a screening trial succeeded on its seventh try.

[‡] Ideally, of course, this will mean *reconvening* the group who met and worked with your mentee in preparing their original grant application.

5 The author's colleagues are divided on whether one should ever appeal a rejection. Most wouldn't, except when there was glaring unfairness or bias.[§]

6 If the agency hasn't included a rating score in their rejection note, mentees should ask them for it. If it's in the fundable range, mentees can take courage and start thinking how to make the application more attractive (more on this later). If it's very low, mentees can get ready for a major revision or submission to a different agency. But they can take courage from the fact that the author has seen the same grant, when submitted to two agencies, receive a terrible score from one and a top score from the other, often as a result of the quality of other grants in the same competition.

7 Mentees can find out the agency's rules about resubmission formats, beginning with the permitted length of the reapplication, whether they allow additional tables and appendices, whether prior scores are admissible (a tough judgment call, which needs thorough discussion with a mentor), whether they permit lengthy covering letters addressing criticisms of the original application, and whether they permit letters of support from institutions or from external content or methods experts who support their study.

8 Mentees should pass whatever they've learned during this initial step along to their R&R team.

C Mentees should then incorporate what they've learned so far into a "hard-nosed" review of their rejected application:

1 Again and again, they should ask themselves (and others) whether their research question [6] was framed in the clearest, most imaginative and exciting way that will engage and enthuse their next round of reviewers.

2 They should assess whether they really made a compelling case for their study. This usually requires updating their literature search, looking for more convincing recent evidence on the burden of the problem they're attacking, the biological–clinical–educational–health-care rationale for their intervention (and its competitors), the clinical equipoise and enthusiasm of potential clinical collaborators and relevant voluntary health organizations, and the societal benefits of gaining a definitive answer to their research question. Because other investigators' citations will speak louder to reviewers than your

---

[§] The authors know of one case in which a successful appeal and rejection-reversal followed exposure of a blatantly sexist review.

mentee's own declarations, they should approach the former for inclusion in their resubmission.

3 Has your mentee's project become more feasible than it appeared at the time of their unsuccessful application? Since then, have they generated any good news about the commitment of their collaborators and institutions, the availability of eligible participants, the practicability of their interventions, the successful testing of their study procedures and data forms, or the precision and accuracy of their outcome measures? Documenting these in your mentee's reapplication will demonstrate that they are continuing to actively pursue their research question, not passively waiting for the reapplication deadline.

4 Should your mentee try to harness (more) public or media support? This strategy could help or backfire, and ought to be discussed with their mentor before proceeding.

5 Mentees should ask themselves whether they've assembled the right team of collaborators for their project. For example, if they propose a statistical analysis but didn't already recruit a statistician co-investigator on their initial application, they should beg forgiveness from one and seek their collaboration from now on.[¶] Are there other content or methods experts who would improve both the quality of their study and its credibility to grant reviewers (especially if their most critical reviewer's discipline isn't already represented in the membership of your mentee's study team)? And if, after helping your mentee, these additional experts can't or won't formally join the study, can your mentee at least get them to write strong letters of support that could be appended to their reapplication?

6 Especially early in their careers, or if this is their first study of this sort, should your mentee recruit a renowned investigator (known and respected by grant reviewers) as a co-principal investigator?[‖]

7 Mentees should identify whether any of their application's criticisms are "false-positives"? That is, are any of the criticized elements of their application scientifically correct, but expressed in so confusing

---

[¶] Some Canadian agencies demand statistician co-investigators on all randomized trials.

[‖] Indeed, since the objective here is to get the money, the author discusses with mentees whether this senior person should be named the principal investigator on the reapplication, as long as there is the prior, written understanding that the mentee trades places with them when it comes to presenting and "lead-authoring" the study's results. This is a judgment call, balancing prospects for funding against the appearance of a lack of independence.

a fashion that reviewers conclude that your mentee is wrong about them? If so, mentees can draft clearer versions and try them out on colleagues until they are readily understood.

8 If the application is for a randomized trial, does your mentee need to rethink its placement along the explanatory–pragmatic continuum?[7] That is, has your mentee jumped too early into asking a lengthy mega-cluster trial *pragmatic* question (e.g. does their intervention work when offered to patients in the hurly-burly of routine health care in multiple centers?) when they'd be better off asking a quicker *explanatory* question (e.g. can their intervention work among previously consenting high-risk, highly responsive patients cared for by expert clinicians) in a single center?

9 Again, for an application to fund a randomized trial, are all the elements of your mentee's protocol consistent with its location along this explanatory–pragmatic continuum? Have they (for example) inserted elaborate compliance measurements, interventions for low compliers, and "per-protocol" analyses in an otherwise highly pragmatic trial?

10 Is obtaining your mentee's primary outcome measure vulnerable to participants becoming lost to follow-up? If so, do they need to search for routine administrative databases that will capture the outcomes of lost participants, or should they be incorporating "stepwise informed de-consent" that permits them to obtain at least the primary outcome measurements on participants who have stopped their assigned interventions and left their study?

11 Has your mentee proposed gathering too much data from too many sources? Are their protocol and data forms morbidly obese with demands for data that are extraneous to their study question? If so, could they be eliminated, or ascertained on only random subsets of participants and visits?

12 As a result of the foregoing, is the agency choking on the size of your mentee's budget (even after they invoked a policy of cutting all budgets by, say, 20%)? How would it look if they progressively eliminated the trimmable fat?

13 But might the agency still choke on your mentee's budget after it has been trimmed? Should they remove some or all of the interesting sub-studies from their reapplication? In the extreme, should your mentee transform their request and only ask for seed money for a pilot study? Alternatively, should they carve up their application and apply for different components of it from different agencies?

14 Along the way, your mentee should make sure they have addressed any other criticisms they've learned from their rejection letter or contact with the agency.

15 Based on all the foregoing, mentees should prepare a master checklist of issues that they think must be dealt with in resurrecting their grant application.

16 Finally, mentees should insert the products of their hard-nosed review as brief notations in their unsuccessful application document (perhaps using their word-processor's "Track Changes" and "New Comments" functions for greater clarity) and send it to you and the other members of their R&R team *before* it meets. Doing so will not only help focus that discussion, but will show them that your mentee is taking the major initiative in resurrecting the application (rather than simply expecting the R&T team to bail you out).

D While waiting for that meeting, your mentee should devote time and energy to their other academic activities (e.g. completing that systematic review that is sitting on their writing desk, polishing off that secondary analysis of their last study, and diversifying other elements of their academic portfolio).

Stage II. The mentee's meeting with their R&R team

1 Mentees should be encouraged to chair the session, deferring to their seniors but keeping them on topic.

2 Mentees can begin with a round-robin so that everybody can express their condolences, identify what they think are the greatest problems with the rejected grant, suggest what can be done to solve them, and publicly state whether/how they will help your mentee rewrite it. Mentees can add these comments and commitments to their master checklist and circulate it around their R&R team.

3 After the round-robin, mentees can raise any remaining items from their master checklist for discussion and resolution.

4 Most importantly, mentees can seek consensus around classifying their application's criticisms into four groups:
  • Group 1: Major problems which must be corrected
  • Group 2: Major problems which cannot be corrected**

** If there are more than two of these, mentees had better reconsider resubmitting this grant to this same agency.

- Group 3: Minor problems which can be corrected
- Group 4: Minor problems which can be ignored.

5   By the conclusion of that R&R meeting, your mentee should have revised their master checklist accordingly, including who will do what about each problem in preparing the resubmission.

Stage III. Re-writing the application

1   Mentees should give themselves plenty of time for the re-write, and their R&R team plenty of time to digest it. Mentees should be brought to recognize that few things will frustrate and turn off an R&R team quicker than being asked to provide comments on their next draft by the next morning. R&R team members both need and deserve time to think and respond thoughtfully.

2   Mentees should avoid the Scylla of telling the agency that their reviewers were stupid, biased, or both (mentees were supposed to have finished with anger and remorse before this stage).

3   Mentees should also avoid the Charybdis of repeatedly thanking the agency and its reviewers for each and every criticism and suggestion in their rejection letter. A single, global, sincere statement of appreciation, noting that their criticisms led to a stronger protocol, will suffice. Mentees need to present themselves as thoughtful investigators who appreciate and respond to constructive criticism, not as fawning toadies.

4   In rewriting their applications, mentees should be sure to address they agency's criticisms as they go. Mentees should tell them what they propose to do to solve the major (Group 1) and minor (Group 3) correctable problems, and why they cannot solve the major uncorrectable (Group 2) problems (especially if they would require a huge increase in the study budget). There is no need to comment on Group 4.

5   Mentees should remember that it is appropriate to challenge a reviewer in a respectful fashion. If a solution they propose for one of the problems is inferior to the one your mentee decides to employ, they should acknowledge that there are different ways to skin that particular cat and justify the way that they've decided to use, citing any literature (including CONSORT [8]) that supports their decision. Along the way, mentees might quietly note when different reviewers disagree with each other.

6   If the agency permits a lengthy covering letter accompanying their resubmission, mentees should begin it with their global thanks and then proceed through their responses to their criticisms in Groups 1–3.

7   Mentees should consider making their referees' second go at the submission easier for them by presenting revisions in a different typeface or as "Track Changes."

8   Of course, mentees should send drafts of the re-submission to their R&R team for additional suggestions and comments.

Stage IV. Re-submission of the application

1   Whenever your mentee, you, and their R&R team are satisfied, or by the agency's deadline, whichever comes first.

Once funded and underway, the inevitable methodological, logistic, inter-personal and (we hope not) financial encountered by the mentee become prime topics for the agenda of subsequent mentorship meetings. When the study is completed, a host of new mentorship challenges arise in writing up, presenting, and publishing its results, and we will take these up in the next chapter.

Bottom line and scenario resolution

Your mentee requires several days to recover from the disappointment and anger following their grant rejection, but has a solid support system and are soon ready for battle. Convinced (and convincing you) that their study wasn't too late, too early, too uninteresting, or too time-consuming to fix, they arm themselves with the strategies and tactics presented in this chapter and get to work. After forming and alerting their R&R team, they contact the agency, confirm that they can reapply, and receive referees' comments (which, although critical and citing the need for additional statistical expertise, encour-age reapplication). They draft a reapplication (using the "Track Changes" and "Comment" functions for the benefit of their busy R&R team), cite promising pilot data they gathered since submitting the original application, recruit a statistical co-PI, tighten the budget, classify the criticisms for importance and correctability and draft responses to them, and send the resulting draft to the R&R team a week before they meet. The meeting goes well – in large part because they chair and control it – and members follow through on their pledges to contribute to the reapplication. After receiving R&R team feed-back on two further drafts, the revised application, accompanied by all the required ethical and institutional permissions, makes it to the agency by the resubmission deadline.

It gets funded this time.

References

1. Straus SE, McAlister FA, Sackett DL, Deeks JJ. The accuracy of patient history, wheezing, and laryngeal measurements in diagnosing obstructive airway disease. CARE-COAD1 Group. Clinical assessment of the reliability of the examination-chronic obstructive airways disease. JAMA 2000; 12: 1853–7.
2. Guyatt G, Sackett D, Taylor DW, *et al*. Determining optimal therapy–randomized trials in individual patients. N Engl J Med 1986; 314: 889–92.

3. National Institutes of Health Website. Grant writing tips sheets. Available at: http://grants.nih.gov/grants/grant_tips.htm. Accessed 25 October 2012.
4. Szatmari P, Sackett DL. Clinician-trialist rounds: 11. When your grant gets turned down – Part 1: Remorse, anger and reconciliation. Clinical Trials J 2012; 9: 447–9.
5. Szatmari P, Sackett DL. Clinician-trialist rounds: 12. When your grant gets turned down – Part 2: Resurrection. Clinical Trials J 2012; 9: 660.
6. Sackett DL. The tactics of performing therapeutic trials. In: Haynes RB, Sackett DL, Guyatt GH, Tugwell P. *Clinical Epidemiology*, 3rd edn. Philadelphia: Lippincott Williams & Wilkins, 2006; pp 72–3.
7. Thorpe KE, Zwarenstein M, Oxman AO, *et al.* A pragmatic-explanatory continuum indicator summary (PRECIS): a tool to help trial designers. J Clin Epid 2009; 62: 464–75.
8. The Consort Statement. Available at: http://www.consort-statement.org/consort -statement/overview0/. Accessed 6 June 2012.

Chapter 4.4 **Some effective mentoring strategies and tactics**

*Part 4: Mentoring for knowledge dissemination**

Scenario

You have meetings with three mentees (a clinician-educator, a biostatistician, and a clinician-scientist) coming up and you just received the agendas that they proposed for these meetings. Each of them has listed under the "High priority" heading a request for help with a talk they are to give at a prestigious meeting next month, including the words: "too many slides?" and "too long?" and "help with hostile questions." The clinician-educator will be presenting the results of his evaluation of a new educational program for undergraduate medical students; the biostatistician will be presenting the evaluation of a statistical approach to multivariate analysis; and the clinician-scientist is presenting preliminary results from a pragmatic randomized trial. Under the "Medium priority" heading one of them has highlighted a manuscript they emailed you about earlier that was rejected by their first choice of journal, along with the annotation: "What do I do now?" You collect your thoughts as to how to respond to these requests.

The generation of new knowledge, while valuable in its own right, benefits neither its targets nor its creator until it is disseminated. This chapter addresses the mentor's role in helping mentees accomplish that dissemination through the spoken and written word. As with research grants, the authors believe that learning how to make audio-visual presentations and how to generate, submit, and resurrect rejected journal manuscripts are such fundamental prerequisites for academic success that they should be taken

---

* This chapter focuses on knowledge dissemination, and we refer readers to other resources for information on knowledge implementation such as: Straus SE, Tetroe J, Graham ID (eds) *Knowledge Translation in Health Care*, 2nd edn. Wiley Blackwell, 2013.

Mentorship in Academic Medicine, First Edition. Sharon E. Straus and David L. Sackett.
© 2014 John Wiley & Sons, Ltd. Published 2014 by John Wiley & Sons, Ltd.

up during mentees' graduate training, and not postponed until they are scrambling to generate first-time presentations and publications as a new postdoc or faculty member. This is also the place to reiterate that the order of authorship of any academic presentation should be set down in writing before submitting the grant proposal for the research that will generate its contents.

Audio-visual presentations

Probably as soon as a research project begins, and certainly when it begins to generate results, mentees will start presenting its protocol and findings in talks accompanied by electronic slides. Because these presentations are "performances" that will make or sometimes break the mentee's reputation, both as a scientist worth respecting and a communicator worth listening to, effective mentors make sure they incorporate the best of both science and "show-biz".

Mentors can help mentees accomplish this by guiding them through the following three steps:

1 The mentee prepares an initial draft of both text and slides, sends them in advance to their mentor, and presents them at a mentorship meeting.

2 The goal of this session is to put the mentee through the most rigorous challenge they will ever face in presenting their work, but in a confidential and safe setting. The mentor provides candid feedback, and is permitted to be quite blunt and highly critical in this one-on-one protected and supportive atmosphere. Criticisms of science include clarity in presenting the study question, methods, results, discussion, threats to validity, implications, and future plans. Criticisms of "show-biz" include dress, body language, voice, speed and clarity of speech, choice of words, sequence of presentation, coordination of speech and slides, slide colors/font size/crowding/building/avoidance of fancy slide changes, and the like. Following the discussion of this feedback, effective mentors pose the most challenging questions and criticisms the mentee will be likely to face following a public presentation.

3 The mentee revises the presentation accordingly and – when both they and their mentor are satisfied with it – presents it again, this time to an invited group of peers and expert faculty, both groups preselected for supportive attitudes toward the mentee's success. Again, feedback is provided on both science and show-biz, and likely questions and criticisms are raised and the most effective responses identified. Again, the objective here is to allow mentees to face the greatest skepticism and toughest challenges at home, among their friends and supporters, rather than at a foreign venue among strangers and rivals.

4 Returning home after the formal presentation, it's useful for the mentor and mentee to debrief after the presentation, not just to review any interesting questions that arose from the audience but also the presentation itself. If the presentation was video-recorded or webcast, they could review that and discuss the effective and less effective aspects of the mentee's voice, gestures, posture, response to questions, etc., identifying the elements they'd like to work on and improve before the next presentation. Alternatively, the mentee could have asked two or three friends in the audience to provide written feedback after the presentation.

Publications

Mentees writing for publication in peer-reviewed journals should already have been introduced to the rigors of getting manuscripts past peer reviewers by having carried out duplicate, blind reviews of manuscripts previously sent their mentors. By having already learned to recognize fatal flaws in the presentation, discussion, and defense of other authors' conclusions, they will have a head start in presenting, discussing, and defending their own. Moreover, they already will have learned about the restrictions (as for length and style) and requirements (as for citations and permissions) of the target journals in which they aspire to publish.

Armed with this foreknowledge, they must then buckle down and write. The authors of this book have never encountered "born writers," nor successful, effective ones who professed that writing was easy (although most found it fun and gratifying). As described in Chapter 4.1 on time management, the successful authors we know set aside, rigorously control, and jealously protect their writing time.

Effective mentors foster and guide budding authors in several ways. We have already noted the importance of providing prior experience in the creation and discussion of duplicate, blind reviews of manuscripts mentors receive, and in the encouragement and monitoring of protected writing time. Mentors who have favorite texts [1] or "how to" books [2] can loan or recommend them to budding authors.

To these we add the setting of mutually agreed quotas of comprehensible words to be submitted before and discussed during tutorial sessions. Depending on mentees' prior experience and first language, these quotas can range from a weekly production and submission of 300 words to a draft of 3000. As with audio-visual presentations, the objective here is to provide rigorous, blunt criticism in a confidential, supportive setting, so that the ultimately submitted manuscript is devoid of easy reasons to reject it. Once a manuscript emerges successfully from this sheltered process, it is ready to receive more widespread informal review by content experts (carefully selected by the mentor) who will provide additional criticisms and suggestions for their corrections in a rigorous but encouraging manner, all the time respecting the ownership and confidentiality of its contents. Sooner or later, the paper is ready for submission to a journal.

We recommend working with the mentee to set deadlines for each stage of this journey to ensure that the paper gets completed in a timely fashion. Threats to the timeline include waiting for feedback from the above-mentioned reviewers and from co-authors. Accordingly, mentees could find it useful to email their reviewers and co-authors with reasonable timelines for their reviews and edits, such as two weeks (i.e. not 24 hours!). Gentle reminders can be sent a few days before these deadlines and, if no response is received, a follow up email can be sent stating that: "The manuscript will be submitted within the next week. If I don't hear further from you I will assume you are okay with the current draft."

Unless academic deadlines (such as promotion) are pending, mentees can be encouraged to aim high in choosing journals for submission, and their identification and readership will often determine how the manuscript is crafted. We typically ask our mentees to rank the top few journals in which they (and their admirers) would be most chuffed to see their paper in print and, after ruling out only those which don't publish on their topic or would never reach their target audience,[†] encourage them to have a go (under the credo that it is better to have a paper rejected by the New England Journal of Medicine than to never have submitted it to them at all). The exponential growth of electronic journals as this book was in preparation virtually guarantees the eventual publication, somewhere, of any scientific paper containing any valid message. Finally, many granting agencies have adopted policies about ensuring research is available in open access journals, and this should be considered in making this selection.

As with grant applications, the average fate of manuscript submissions to top scientific journals is rejection of the initial submission. Effective mentors prepare their mentees for this rejection and guide them in responding to it. This process is closely similar to that of resurrecting its parent research grant application, the success of which led to the generation of its contents and conclusions. Mentors can help their mentees start this process by encouraging them, first of all, to decide whether their manuscript ought to be resurrected. Of course, the chances of getting it published are now better if the rejection

---

[†] When a paper's content and conclusions are aimed toward readerships with limited funds, we advocate away from avaricious journals with access fees and toward public access (but indexed) publications.

letter told them what their reviewers were thinking. But does the mentee really have a chance to get them to turn their thinking around? The grounds for abandoning the manuscript are three:

1 Is the study they're reporting too *late*? Did their rejection provide convincing evidence that somebody else has beaten your mentee to the punch and already answered their question? 2. Is the study they proposed *too early*?

2 Did their manuscript receive a ghastly rating for a *fatal flaw* that they simply cannot fix?

3 Would it take *too much of their time* away from worthier pursuits to fix this manuscript? Has the parent project lost its scientific value and attractiveness to your mentee in the interim, replaced by a more important and exciting research result that would be far more deserving of their time and effort?

If the manuscript they submitted wasn't too late, too uninteresting, or too time-consuming to fix, it's time to help your mentee convert their distress at its rejection into positive efforts to resurrect and resubmit it. The following paragraphs summarize the parallels to repairing and resubmitting an unsuccessful research grant proposals [3].

The resurrection process occurs in four stages. Along the way, mentees can be encouraged to take comfort in the fact that many seasoned investigators and authors consider getting a paper published a two-stage process, with stage one ending in a rejected manuscript.

Stage I. Steps to take *before* mentees meet with colleagues who can help them

A Mentees should alert their mentor, and anybody else they want to involve in their revision and resubmission team (the "R&R team"), and schedule an urgent meeting with them.[‡] In the meanwhile, mentees should do the following homework:

B Mentees should get as much feedback as possible from the journal. So that they gain both experience and confidence, mentees should ask for help from their mentors only if absolutely necessary.

   1 Is this the mentee's second or greater rejection of this same manuscript? If this is the second rejection by the same journal, it's probably time to move to the next journal on their preferred list.

[‡] Ideally, of course, this will mean *reconvening* the group who met and worked with your mentee in preparing their original manuscript.

2 If their manuscript never got as far as peer review, but was rejected on an initial screen, mentees can try to find out why, although in our experience, detailed information is not usually available at this stage when sought from editors. On the other hand, some journals permit appeals from rejected authors, and it can't hurt to ask whether this is permitted.

3 Most journals nowadays conduct "open" reviews that name the reviewers. This permits mentees to determine their disciplines and judge whether they were appropriate.

4 Most rejection letters indicate whether they want the author to simply go away or are willing to look at a resubmission. In the latter case they typically offer detailed shortcomings and criticisms that must be corrected before they would re-consider publishing it. Responding appropriately to these criticisms is central to any resubmission.

5 Mentees can find out the journal's rules about the resubmission format, the permitted length of a resubmission, whether portions of the paper should be resubmitted as appendices, and how the letter accompanying the resubmission should address criticisms of the original manuscript.

6 Mentees should pass whatever they've learned during this initial step along to their R&R team.

C Mentees should then incorporate what they've learned so far into a "hard-nosed" review of their rejected manuscript:

1 Again and again, they should ask themselves (and others) whether the underlying theme of their manuscript was framed in the clearest, most imaginative and exciting way that would engage and enthuse their next round of reviewers.

2 They should assess whether they really made a compelling case for their study and its conclusions. This usually requires updating their literature search, looking for more convincing recent evidence on the burden of the problem they're describing, the biological–clinical–educational–health-care rationale for their thesis, and the health-care and societal benefits of their conclusions.

3 Has their paper become more relevant and important than it appeared at the time of their unsuccessful submission? Since then, has the appearance of other publications raised the relevance and importance of their paper? Documenting these in your mentee's reapplication will demonstrate that they are continuing to actively pursue their research area and are keeping up to date.

4 Mentees should ask themselves whether they've assembled the right team of co-authors. For example, if they conducted a complex statistical

analysis but didn't include a statistician co-author, they should and seek their collaboration now and decide whether further analyses would strengthen the paper. Are there other content or methods experts who would improve both the quality and credibility of the manuscript (especially if their most critical reviewer's discipline wasn't already represented in the authorship of the unsuccessful manuscript)?

5 Is the credibility of the manuscript vulnerable to participants becoming lost to follow-up? If so, do they need to search for routine administrative databases that will capture the outcomes of lost participants and update their analysis?

6 Along the way, your mentee should make sure they have addressed any other criticisms they've learned from their rejection letter or contact with the journal.

7 Some research centers employ copyeditors to help authors "clarify" their messages. Dave Sackett thinks they depersonalize and corrupt his writing and avoids them, but mentees might want to explore what they might contribute to their own manuscripts.

8 Based on all the foregoing, mentees should prepare a master checklist of issues that they think must be dealt with in resurrecting their manuscript.

9 Finally, mentees should insert the products of their hard-nosed review as brief notations in their unsuccessful manuscript (perhaps using their word-processor's "Track Changes" and "New Comments" functions for greater clarity) and send it to the members of their R&R team *before* it meets. Doing so will not only help focus that discussion, but will show them that your mentee is taking the major initiative in resurrecting the manuscript (rather than simply expecting the R&T team to bail them out).

D While waiting for that meeting, your mentee should devote time and energy to their other academic activities (e.g., completing that systematic review that is sitting on their writing desk, polishing off that secondary analysis of their last study, and diversifying other elements of their academic portfolio).

Stage II. The mentee's meeting with their R&R team

1 Mentees should be encouraged to chair the session, deferring to their seniors but keeping them on topic.

2 Mentees can begin with a round-robin so that their co-authors and other R&R members can express their condolences, identify what they think are the greatest problems with the rejected manuscript, suggest what can

be done to solve them, and publicly state whether/how they will help your mentee rewrite it. Mentees can add these comments and commitments to their master checklist and circulate it around their R&R team.

3 After the round-robin, mentees can raise any remaining items from their master checklist for discussion and resolution.

4 Most importantly, mentees can seek consensus around classifying their paper's criticisms into four groups:

Group 1: Major problems which must be corrected.
Group 2: Major problems which cannot be corrected.
Group 3: Minor problems which can be corrected.
Group 4: Minor problems which can be ignored.

5 By the conclusion of that R&R meeting, your mentee should have revised their master checklist accordingly, including who will do what about each problem in preparing the manuscript revision. Ultimately, however, it is the mentee's responsibility to ensure the manuscript is revised appropriately, and they must take "ownership" of this process.

Stage III. Re-writing the paper

1 Mentees should give themselves plenty of time for the re-write, and their R&R team plenty of time to digest it. Mentees should be brought to recognize that few things will frustrate and turn off an R&R team quicker than being asked to provide comments on their next draft by the next morning. R&R team members both need and deserve time to think and respond thoughtfully.

2 Mentees should avoid the Scylla of telling the journal that their reviewers were stupid, biased, or both.

3 Mentees should also avoid the Charybdis of repeatedly thanking the journal and its reviewers for each and every criticism and suggestion in their rejection letter. A single, global, sincere statement of appreciation, noting that their criticisms led to a stronger manuscript, will suffice.

4 In rewriting their paper, mentees should be sure to address the journal's criticisms as they go. Moreover, if the journal permits a covering letter accompanying their resubmission, mentees should begin it with their global thanks and then proceed through their responses to their criticisms in Groups 1–3. Mentees should tell them how they solved the major (Group 1) and minor (Group 3) correctable problems, and why they cannot solve the major uncorrectable (Group 2) problems. There may be no need to comment on Group 4.

5 Of course, mentees should send redrafts of the manuscript to their R&R team for additional suggestions and comments.

Stage IV: Resubmission

Mentors should monitor the foregoing so that resubmission occurs as swiftly as the foregoing steps permit, both to prevent getting "scooped" by other papers on the same subject and to remind the journal of the conscientious and concerted efforts of the lead author. One of our heroes, Tom Chalmers, when submitting a previously unsuccessful manuscript to a new journal, used to report his failure with a previous one. Sharon Straus has met with success by expanding this tactic to include the previous journal's reviews.

A note on abstracts submitted to scientific meetings

Abstracts for scientific meetings can usefully be regarded as early drafts of the "Summary" for the later definitive manuscript on the same topic. In helping mentees prepare them, mentors should point out that tendering abstracts to scientific meetings differs from submitting papers to refereed journals in six important ways, and can be a two-edged sword:

1 and 2 The first pair of ways describes a paradox: on the one hand, abstracts get just one chance at acceptance, and cannot be revised and resubmitted. On the other hand, the bar is usually set much lower for the publication of meeting abstracts than for the publication of journal articles, so the chances for a submitted abstract appearing in a meetings "Proceedings" range from "high" to "guaranteed," the latter especially for meetings that include poster sessions.

3 At some meetings, abstracts compete for prestigious oral presentations, and in these cases deserve considerably more attention in their preparation, going through repeated cycles of in-house submission, criticism, and revision.

4 Accepted abstracts can be added to the mentee's CV, indicating promising scholarly activity. Lots of abstracts suggest lots of promising activity.

5 However, abstracts carry much, much less weight in a CV than refereed publications.

6 Furthermore, abstracts indicate the mere promise of academic success, not its achievement. The latter is found in refereed publications in top journals. Thus, the second edge of the abstract sword can inflict lethal damage to a CV (and the academic career of its owner) if repeated abstracts fail to reappear as refereed publications within the next two to three years.

7 Once established in a research field, most academics divert their precious writing time energies from abstracts to formal manuscripts, except when they have some "hot" ideas or results and want to rapidly disseminate them.

A third strategy for knowledge dissemination employs social media such as Twitter and Facebook, and researchers and research groups are increasingly using these strategies both to disseminate their work[§] and to follow and interact with other researchers. There is a large volume of literature on this topic, but much of it is descriptive and there are no randomized trials of the impact of this dissemination strategy.[¶] Certainly these tools can allow the mentee to develop connections with colleagues around the world without ever meeting them in person, and therefore can help them develop their own professional networks. However, these tools can become as addictive as email, and can easily consume time and energy better spent on other activities. So, as in other aspects of time-management, mentors have to help mentees strike a productive balance.

Teaching

Agreeing with Albert Einstein ("all physical theories, their mathematical expressions apart ought to lend themselves to so simple a description 'that even a child could understand them.'" [4]), Ernest Rutherford ("A theory that you can't explain to a bartender is probably no damn good." [5]) and Kurt Vonnegut Jr's Felix Hoenikker ("Dr. Hoenikker used to say that any scientist who couldn't explain to an eight-year-old what he was doing was a charlatan." [6]) we hold that the best teachers are *not* the ones who *know* more than anybody else, but the ones who can *explain* what they *do* know *to* anybody else. We claim support for this position from the contemporaneous literature generated by "real" educationalists, who have kindly introduced us to several excellent resources [7, 8, 9, 10, 11].

Thus, effective teaching is more the product of skills than of knowledge (as long as the latter is current), and effective mentors put their mentees into situations in which they can observe skilled teachers, gain teaching skills, and be observed in their application of these teaching skills.

Phase 1 places mentees where they can observe ("shadow") role-model teachers in relevant settings, addressing relevant matters. For academic clinicians this usually involves two placements, one in the clinical settings where the mentee aspires to become an excellent inpatient or outpatient clinical teacher, and the second in the class- or seminar-room where the

---

[§] They should determine whether reporting their results on social media jeopardizes publication in their target print journal.
[¶] Lisa Hartling (from the University of Alberta) is leading a knowledge synthesis of the impact of social media on behavior change and the results from this will be available in 2013.

mentee aspires to become an excellent teacher of content or methods. The mentee's objective is the identification and discussion of effective teaching and evaluation methods by a role model, and often this is best and most efficiently provided by their mentor.

If not their mentor, the selection of appropriate role models to shadow is paramount. Regardless of their seniority, we advise against placement with teachers who aggressively interrogate individual learners with progressively challenging questions of fact until the latter collapse (a strategy labelled "pimping" [12]), for that is bullying, not teaching. Rather, placement should seek teachers whose non-threatening style and employment of problem-solving tactics help learners reason through a patient's predicament or an issue in content or methods.

In Phase 2, and by agreement with their role-model teachers, mentees change roles with them and lead portions of the educational events, followed by private discussions around what worked and didn't work and how the mentee's performance could become more effective. The unobtrusive videotaping of relevant sessions can provide a rich set of observations for discussion and remediation. This phase continues until both are satisfied that all relevant learning situations have been experienced and evaluated.

Once mentees become independent teachers, and by mutual consent, they take over the sessions, and mentors can attend and later offer feedback around their teaching strategies and tactics. Some universities have established formal teaching consultation services that may also help a mentee refine their teaching technique.[||]

A worthy secondary outcome of all the foregoing processes is the mentee's development of mentoring skills so that they can, in turn, become mentors themselves. Once mentees become independent teachers, and by mutual consent, mentors can attend their teaching sessions, followed by exchanges over teaching strategies and tactics.

Bottom line and scenario resolution

You review your mentees' first sets of slides and each of them has included too much information on a single slide that can't be read from beyond the first row (for example, the clinician-scientist has included the trial design on a single slide). You've also found that:
* the clinician-educator has included too much animation in the slide deck which distracts from their excellent scholarly work

---

[||] For example, the Stanford University Center for Teaching and Learning. See http://ctl.stanford.edu/about/mission.html. Accessed 8 January 2013.

- the biostatistician has included too many formulae which you fear will not be understandable to the largely clinical audience she will be addressing
- the clinician-scientist has included too many cartoons that distract from the message and lengthen the talk.

You meet with each of the mentees to review their slides. Each is relieved that you can trash them in private. Posing (in the nastiest way) what you reckon are the most challenging questions they'll face, you send your mentees away to revise and rearm. They email a revised and much improved slide set and present their talk to a "friendly" audience of fellow mentees and faculty. Acting on the additional suggestions and challenges they receive there, they return from their out-of-town formal presentation quite chuffed at their reception, and get down to writing up the research project for publication.

Alas, the resulting manuscript is refused by the mentee's journal of choice, but by applying the strategies described in this chapter, and encouraged by one of their reviewers, they succeed with a revised manuscript.

Along the way, each of the mentees "shadow" you as you teach – both at the bedside and in the classroom – and gradually develop their own, effective, and popular didactic style.

References

1. For example, Strunk W Jr,, White EB, Angell R. *The Elements of Style*, 4th edn. Boston: Allyn & Bacon, 2000.
2. For example, Silva PJ. *How to Write a Lot: A Practical Guide of Productive Academic Writing*. Washington: American Psychological Association, 2007.
3. Szatmari P, Sackett DL. Clinician-trialist rounds: 12. When your grant gets turned down – Part 2: Resurrection. Clin Trials J 2013 (in press).
4. DeBroglie L. *New Perspectives in Physics*. New York: Basic Books, Inc; p. 184.
5. Collins FS. *The Language of God: A Scientist Presents Evidence for Belief*. New York: Free Press – Simon and Schuster, 2006; p. 60.
6. Vonnegut K Jr. *Cat's Cradle*. New York: Dell Publishing Co, Inc; 1963, p. 32.
7. Davis BG. *Tools for Teaching*. 2nd end. San Francisco: John Wiley & Sons, 2009.
8. Ambrose SA, Bridges MW, DiPietro M, Lovett MC, Norman MK. *How Learning Works: Seven Research-based Principles for Smart Teaching*. San Francisco: John Wiley & Sons, 2010.
9. Dornan T, Mann KV, Scherpbier AJJA, Spencer JA (eds). *Medical Education: Theory and Practice*. Edinburgh: Churchill Livingstone, 2011.
10. Swanwick T (ed). *Understanding Medical Education: Evidence, Theory and Practice*. Oxford: Wiley-Blackwell, 2010.
11. Skeff K. Analyzing the complex task of teaching. Available at: http://www.stanford.edu/dept/CTL/AWT/Skeff_99.html. Accessed Feb 2013.
12. Detsky AS. The art of pimping. JAMA. 2009; 301: 1379–81.

Chapter 4.5   Some effective mentoring strategies and tactics

Part 5: Mentoring for promotion, protection, and job prospects

Mentees' victories in meeting and overcoming the challenges presented in the preceding four chapters will determine both their academic "success" (promotion, tenure, and the like) and their quality of life (work–life balance, satisfaction, happiness). There remain six areas in which mentors play vital roles in these victories.

1. The timely achievement of milestones in mentees' academic progress

Effective mentors help their mentees keep an eye on the academic calendar, setting and monitoring targets for accomplishing crucial milestones such as winning their MSc and/or PhD degrees. Of key importance here is "backward planning" of the elements of this success:
- by what date should the required and elective courses be completed?
- by what date should a thesis topic be determined and a thesis committee formed?
- by what date should a first draft of the thesis be circulated?

  This same approach can be used for other milestones such as obtaining a first operating grant or career investigator award. Achieving these targets on time gives the mentee a positive reputation as a "finisher". Failing to meet them on time risks creating a negative reputation as "disorganized" or a "non-finisher". The differential effects of these reputations on a mentee's subsequent academic advancement and life-satisfaction are profound.

2. Creation and maintenance of an effective curriculum vitae

Effective mentors help their mentees create and especially maintain CVs that not only document their accomplishments but present them to prospective employers as highly productive and accomplished. This begins by providing

Mentorship in Academic Medicine, First Edition. Sharon E. Straus and David L. Sackett.
© 2014 John Wiley & Sons, Ltd. Published 2014 by John Wiley & Sons, Ltd.

mentees with a template (usually a version suggested by their university) and a sample CV from a successful academic a few years senior to them. Mentees then draft and submit their own at mentoring meetings, receiving feedback on its iterations. Beginning at once, mentees are reminded to add all relevant activities and accomplishments to their growing CV. Indeed, one element they may wish to consider in deciding whether to take on a short-term task is how it would add depth and breadth to their CV. In doing so, their contributions should be clearly stated, but never exaggerated (exposure of exaggerated or false accomplishments destroys the credibility of the real ones). Success in this tedious but vital task is measured by a mentee's ability to polish and fire it off on the same day that they are nominated for an award or offered a job.

3. Creation and maintenance of an effective teaching dossier

Maintaining a detailed record of every teaching contribution is also vital element of academic advance. We recommend this start when a mentee is still a trainee, both to capture early teaching contributions and to perfect the organization of the dossier; it is between difficult and impossible to recreate this summary of teaching activities retrospectively, several years down the career path at promotion time. Different universities have different requirements for a teaching dossier (and we encourage mentees to attend local workshops on developing CVs and teaching dossiers if they are available). If they aren't, mentees' documentation of teaching events should at least record:
- the type of teaching session (i.e. small group, large group, individual)
- the learners (i.e. number of learners and their stage: undergraduate, postgraduate, graduate, or continuing education)
- the setting (i.e. local, national, international)
- all evaluations of their performance and effectiveness (e.g. teaching effectiveness scores and other evaluation metrics).

4. Protection from sharks

The authors have worked at nine universities in five countries on three continents. At each of them, we encountered some outstanding faculty with whom it was a joy to teach, learn, and commune. However, at each of them we also encountered a few predatory faculty who exploited, stole ideas from, back-stabbed, and/or publicly humiliated their juniors. Richard Johns has appropriately labeled them "sharks," and the six rules he laid down for how to swim with them should be mastered by anyone considering an academic career [1]:

1 *Assume unidentified fish are sharks* (until you see them behave kindly in the presence of a shark-attack).
2 *Do not bleed* (by publicly displaying dismay or defeat when attacked by a shark).
3 *Counter any aggression promptly* (early on, by reporting them to your mentor; later, by challenging their first, tentative aggression).
4 *Get out if someone is bleeding* (to avoid becoming a second target).
5 *Use anticipatory retaliation* (remind them at intervals that you won't stand for any repetition of their bad behavior).
6 *Disorganize an organized attack* (by either redirecting their aggression toward other sharks or by introducing something so outrageous that they become disorganized).

In addition to "inoculating" mentees by suggesting that they study Prof. Johns' rules and by pointing out the local sharks, effective mentors not only insist that their mentees report any shark attacks, but also vigorously apply rules #3 and #5 to the offending elasmobranch. In the case of idea-theft, referral to the relevant ombudsman or chair should immediately follow. In the others, face-to-face confrontation by the mentor or a more senior designee can be effective (for example, on two occasions, Dave Sackett prevented further attacks by employing the language of a longshoreman and threatening to throw the offender down a stairwell for any repeat offense).

5. Getting the right next job

Effective mentors play a major role in helping mentees obtain "dream jobs." Their help occurs in three phases: exposure, exploration, and expedition.

Exposure

Exposure begins early in a mentorship, and is accomplished by introducing their mentees to outstanding prospective employers whose ideas, environments, and track records for promoting and protecting newcomers make them ideal individuals to whom to pass the mentoring torch. These introductions can be initiated at scientific meetings, and reinforced by inviting the prospective employers back home for visiting professorships that include social events and individual interviews as well as scientific sessions. When the foregoing is geographically impossible (as when Sharon Straus's mentor in Toronto wanted to introduce her to Dave Sackett in Oxford) the introduction has to occur electronically or on paper.

Exploration

If both parties become seriously interested in linking up, effective mentors then explore the prospective move from both sides. This begins by examining the particulars of the job offer: exactly what sorts of opportunities (including space, support staff, and start-up funds) and obligations (especially the allocation and protection of time for research and writing) are – or need to be – spelled out? What is the academic level of the appointment, and what are the ground rules and expectations of the associated university or research center? Is a formal mentoring system in place at the new institution? The mentor's exploration then moves to other areas: What is the track record of other recruits who have gone before? What do other candid contacts have to say about the prospective employer and environment?

Effective mentors also explore their mentee's understanding of, and attitudes toward, the job on offer. The key element here is helping the mentee distinguish between wanting to be wanted for this job (Who wouldn't? It's very flattering to be offered most jobs) and wanting to actually do this job (Does it really fit their priority lists, will it advance their primary career objectives, is it a nice place to live, etc.?). Because the wages of confusing the former for the latter are so large (lost time, low productivity, family disruption, and burnout) it's crucial to sort this out before accepting the appointment.*

Expedition

Effective mentors will already have made sure that their mentee's CV – vital to the prospective employer's appointments process – is both impressive and accurate. Helping their mentee draft their negotiating letters and respond to the new institution's replies can avoid misunderstandings and document the promises from both sides, should the need arise to refer back to them later. In this negotiating process, mentees should be constantly reminded that, when receiving an invitation to take on a new post, "the invitees' best offer is their first offer", and that all essential resources need to be guaranteed in writing in advance.

Once the hard bargaining is completed, mentors can send letters of introduction to their other friends at the new institution, asking them to introduce themselves and make their new colleague welcome, thereby helping to establish a friendly, nurturing new home. Making sure their mentee is connected to appropriate real estate expertise is also valuable.

---

* When one of her mentees was considering a job at another university, Sharon Straus was asked by their division director, Alun Edwards, to become the "agent" for this mentee, participating in the job discussions as her mentee's advocate. With her mentee's agreement, Sharon accepted this role.

Once their mentee takes up their new post, effective mentors keep in touch, seeking that fine balance between over-involvement and neglect.

6. Deciding when a mentee should become a mentor

Most mentees already provide some elements of mentorship to their contemporaries and more junior trainees (such as on clinical teams). However, as their careers progress and they receive faculty appointments, they need to decide when to take on "formal" mentees. We suggest that they consider:

1 Focusing their first three faculty years on their own careers, ensuring that they establish their own, unique niches. They can start participating on thesis committees, but we recommend against taking primary supervisor roles until they've participated in the complete thesis process for at least one person (beside themselves!). Similarly, we advise against becoming a formal mentor of junior faculty at this early stage, not only because they won't yet have the professional networks or experience to help a mentee, but also because, if the prospective mentee is also in their same research area, competition for ideas and resources may become untenable.

2 Attending a mentorship workshop. These workshops can help clarify the program requirements as well as providing resources for mentorship support.

3 And, when they do take on their first mentee, starting with just one and not taking on a second until the first is well-established.

A role-model mentor

We close this series of chapters with one of Dave Sackett's former graduate students and current colleagues, who kindly permitted us to describe her mentoring activities in detail. Dr Dianne Bryant, a mid-career PhD health researcher, tenured associate professor, is engaged in a broad, multimillion-dollar array of collaborative clinical (rehabilitation and surgery) and health care research, is the director of a data management company, and teaches at the undergraduate and graduate levels. Outside of work, she is a mother of two young children, chauffeur, homework supervisor and tutor, bookkeeper, housekeeper, and groundskeeper; manager of a children's international preparatory choir, book club member, and boot camp enthusiast.

Lest any readers judge the breadth and depth of the mentoring activities described in this book to be beyond the capabilities of any single individual, we offer Dr Bryant's responses to our survey questionnaire in the following appendix.

Appendix A: Dr. Bryant's responses to our survey questionnaire

Item: Developing optimal interactions with their mentor

What tactic(s) have you developed to meet this target?

1 Establish the ground rules – write a contract between mentee and mentor that outlines the responsibilities of each including administrative details (e.g. how to book meetings). This document is actually circulated by our graduate student office to all supervisors and students (usually around September or as part of the student's orientation package) and we are encouraged to review them and sign them with our students (few do, unfortunately).

2 Graduate student group meetings versus individual sessions – I hold monthly meetings with all of my graduate students together (and sometimes the graduate students of close colleagues), where each student updates me on the status of their project, any problems, solutions (if we need a solution, we discuss it as a group), we discuss whether we need to bring in another expert, etc.; we discuss vacations or conflicts in time, whether students can help each other out, etc. The second half of the meeting is spent discussing a common topic (e.g. informed consent, writing the ethics application, scientific writing, how to construct a case report form, database development, SPSS, how to operate the statistical package, etc.) – things they all need but don't get from their course work.

3 Each meeting a student is appointed to takes the minutes of each the meeting we have and circulates them to member attendees before they are finalized. This keeps us all straight (me especially) on decisions, action items and deadlines. I then use this document to add items to my calendar so that I can keep my end of the bargain.

What are the limitations of this tactic?
- 1, 2, and 3 – I haven't found any.

What was the impact of applying these tactics?
- 2 and 3 have positively impacted my efficiency and effectiveness – 1 and 3 have positively impacted transparency and clarity.

Item: Developing effective time-management skills

What tactic(s) have you developed to meet this target?
- During student group meetings when each student is presenting their progress, problems, etc., we take this opportunity to re-identify the goals, discuss next steps, and to prioritize the remaining tasks – to de-mystify

some of the tasks or break them down into manageable chunks (that helps them to get done sometimes); all students are encouraged to share their ideas for managing problems.

What are the strengths of this tactic?

- Students learns to identify tasks, assess their importance in terms of reaching the end goal, which makes the task of prioritizing easier.

What was the impact of applying these tactics?

- Removing the feeling of being overwhelmed.
- Learning that it is okay to say no.
- Learning to decide what to say no to.

Item: Achieving an optimal work/life balance

What tactic(s) have you developed to meet this target?

1 I share my strategy of setting aside writing time, email time, home time (i.e. *no* email or work during family time – turn off the Blackberry), extracurricular activities, saying "no" (how to do it, how do I decide what to say no to, how does this change as I move through my career).

2 Asking the students during our group sessions to share their strategies.

3 Asking the students during our group sessions to share situations where they are encountering difficulty - share our experiences.

What are the strengths of this tactic?

- It gives the student permission (if they need it) to develop a similar strategy; the student can see that a strategy is a necessary component of success.

What are the limitations of this tactic?

- I haven't found any.

What was the impact of applying these tactics?

- Development of a stronger collegial relationship – that I'm not superior to them (for some reason some come in thinking that way) but rather just further along in my career; encourages openness, honesty, respect for family/downtime (your own and that of others); reduced stress levels.

Item: Becoming effective members (and eventual leaders) of research teams

What tactic(s) have you developed to meet this target?

- Modeling and encouraging the attitude of inclusivity.
- Emphasizing the importance of the team.

What are the strengths of this tactic?

- Valuation for the expertise of others; not feeling like you have to do it all yourself or that not being able to do it all yourself is somehow a weakness.

What are the limitations of this tactic?
- The larger the team, the more difficult it is to function in terms of organizing meetings, reaching agreements, etc. It can take a while to demonstrate that taking a little longer with the right team will result in a superior end product than a quicker result that was missing content.

Item: Maximizing their grant success (in preparation, presentation, and response to reviews)
What tactic(s) have you developed to meet this target?

   1 The student is asked to draft the grant; we use serial methods of reviewing to improve the grant.
   2 Share examples of successful and unsuccessful grants.
   3 Teach diplomacy when responding to reviewers.
   4 Demonstrate a method for response.
   5 Rephrase of comment with a clear concise response.
   6 Can you respond to all comments or (because of space restrictions) must you select a few comments to respond to, etc.?

What are the strengths of this tactic?
- Practical hands on experience.

What are the limitations of this tactic?
- Depending on the student (writing skills, ability to summarize, etc.) this can take longer than doing it yourself.

What was the impact of applying these tactics?
- Student gains confidence in grant writing.

Item: Becoming effective and efficient reviewers of grants and papers
What tactic(s) have you developed to meet this target?
- When I receive a request from a journal to serve as a reviewer, I post the requests to review to students who have a similar topic area (content or method) and ask whether they are interested in reviewing the manuscript; they review it independently from me and then we meet together to review the paper and their responses (structure, format, diplomacy).

What are the strengths of this tactic?
- Practical hands on experience.

What are the limitations of this tactic?
- Too many reviews can eat up too much time. I limit the number of reviews I am willing to undertake to about 6 per year and select manuscripts that are close to my expertise so that I reduce or remove the need to spend time refreshing or learning relevant content.

What was the impact of applying these tactics?
- Student gains confidence in reviewing manuscripts.
- Student gains skills in writing their own manuscripts.

Item: Maximizing their writing quality and productivity (including interactions with peer reviewers and editors)

What tactic(s) have you developed to meet this target?

1 I ask that students format their thesis as a manuscript instead of a traditional thesis format.

2 I set a goal that the student submit their thesis for publication at the time they hand in their revised thesis (post defense).

3 I often host group projects – like systematic reviews or methodological projects – that I open up to them (at student group meetings). They are free to participate or not without consequence. We define roles and authorship before beginning the project. Since these projects are outside of their thesis work, it isn't a requirement but an opportunity.

What are the strengths of this tactic?

1 Productivity – mine and theirs.

2 Practical experience for the student (usually with a research design different from their current thesis work).

What are the limitations of this tactic?

1 Sometimes too many students want to be involved. Roles and authorship become important to define a priori.

2 Sometimes students graduate and move on before the project ends – can be difficult to complete.

What was the impact of applying these tactics?
- Students with stronger CVs than those encouraged to only complete their thesis (they often leave with 3–4 publications after an MSc rather than none or one, which is typical for an MSc, and 10 or more as a PhD student).

Item: Becoming effective presenters and speakers (including A-V proficiency)

What tactic(s) have you developed to meet this target?

1 Student prepares their presentation.

2 We hold a mock defense or mock presentation.

3 All my students are asked to attend, and I can usually gather a few faculty members to attend.

4 Following the presentation, the other students offer their comments for improvement, complements and ask questions followed by myself and other faculty.

5 We work on formulating responses in an appropriate tone and mannerism and agree on formulating a concise response if that's needed.

What are the strengths of this tactic?

1 A lot of the time we have 'guessed' the questions that the audience/examiner asks will ask, so the student is well prepared.

2 The student has more confidence in their presentation (as does their supervisor).

What are the limitations of this tactic?
• Time.
What was the impact of applying these tactics?
• Student gains confidence.

Item: Becoming effective classroom and bedside teachers
What tactic(s) have you developed to meet this target?

1 I mentor high school co-op students, MSc and PhD students. I often pair the PhD students with the high school students to act as a mentor. The graduate student participates in educating the high school student on the anatomy, physiology of the injury related to their graduate thesis; prepares the high school student for the operating room; the high school student shadows the graduate student in clinic conducting their research; basically, the graduate student is the high school student's first point of contact for some of their learning.

2 The graduate student drafts some of the student feedback.

3 I have conversations with the graduate student about their experiences (difficulties, successes, etc.).

What are the strengths of this tactic?
• Practical experience teaching and mentoring.
What are the limitations of this tactic?
• I haven't identified any.
What was the impact of applying these tactics?

1 Graduate student gains experience in teaching and mentoring.

2 High school student exposed to cutting edge research, clinical applicability, etc.

Item: Avoiding repeated failure to keep scheduled mentoring meetings

1 Schedule regular meetings well in advance with a start and an end time that are both respected. This is part of the agreement between student and supervisor that we sign at the beginning of each year.

2 Identify when we need a face-to-face meeting versus an email versus an informal five-minute drop-in.

3 Identify tools to facilitate communication to reduce the number of meetings (e.g. student group meetings for common issues (described above) to reduce the number of one-on-one meetings where the content of the meeting is similar between students.

Item: Avoiding failure of either party to follow-through on completing agreed-upon mentoring tasks on time

1 Minutes taken and circulated after each meeting.

2 Agenda with previous minutes attached well before next scheduled meeting, with action items summarized and assigned.

Item: When mentors insist upon lead authorship of papers (or grants) when their mentees have done the lion's share of the intellectual and practical work

Authorship needs to be agreed upon before entering into the relationship and should be a deciding factor in the student choosing that person to be their mentor.

References

1. Johns RJ. Dinner address. How to swim with sharks: the advanced course. Trans Assoc Am Physicians. 1975; 88: 44–54.

Chapter 5 How can you assess, diagnose, and treat mentorship that is in trouble?

Scenario

The mentorship program in your department has been a huge success, judging by the productivity, academic success, and personal satisfaction of both your mentees and mentors. However, there have been occasional problems in the behavior of both mentees and mentors, and your chair has talked you into becoming the official "ombudsperson" for the program.

Your inaugural case-load includes the following:

1 repeated unexplained no-shows at scheduled mentorship meetings by two mentees and two mentors
2 repeated failure of a mentee to complete agreed upon tasks between sessions
3 a case in which mentoring meetings have simply stopped happening
4 a complaint from a mentee that his research interests have been subverted to serve those of his mentor
5 a charge from a mentee that her mentor insisted on lead authorship on a paper describing research into the mentee's original idea and in which she had done most of the work
6 a charge from a mentee that his mentor stole his research idea
7 a complaint from a mentee that they are being bullied by their mentor
8 a charge from a mentee that she has been sexually harassed by her mentor
9 a concern from a mentor that his mentee does not respond to his feedback or suggestions
10 a rumor that one of your mentor–mentee dyads are living together.

How (on earth!) should you handle these cases?

To this point, we have discussed the strategies and tactics that effective mentors and effective mentees can employ to achieve the latters' academic success. Their execution assumes that both members of the dyad are behaving professionally, appropriately, responsibly, and honestly.

Mentorship in Academic Medicine, First Edition. Sharon E. Straus and David L. Sackett.
© 2014 John Wiley & Sons, Ltd. Published 2014 by John Wiley & Sons, Ltd.

Alas, that is not always the case. Accordingly, this chapter addresses the symptoms of mentorships in trouble, identifies their most likely diagnoses, and proposes a range of preventive, curative, and rehabilitative interventions (including, as a last resort, euthanasia). The material in this chapter was identified through our review of the literature (as outlined in Chapter 1), our survey of colleagues, and our own experiences.

Trouble from failing to meet or failing to meet agreements

The first cluster of symptoms of dysfunctional mentorship surrounds mentoring meetings.

Scheduled mentoring meeting no-shows

Because emergencies and other unavoidable interruptions are part of the life of busy academic clinicians, we expect and excuse sporadic no-shows by both mentees and mentors, especially if forewarned and immediately rescheduled to be held soon. However, if they are common, unannounced, and without attempts to reschedule, the mentorship is in trouble.

We suggest that the proper response is for the "innocent" member to insist on meeting to explore possible diagnoses. Does the timing of meetings interfere with the non-attender's child-care responsibilities or other non-negotiable clinical or academic schedules? Are their current format, style, or content irrelevant or otherwise unhelpful to the non-attender? Is too much or too little review of the non-attender's concerns and accomplishments occurring? Has the non-attender fallen out of "like" with the other(s) in the mentorship? Is the non-attender finding better mentoring elsewhere? Does the mentor have too many mentees to be able to make the appropriate commitments to each of them?*

Depending on the diagnosis, changes in the scheduling, format, content, and style of mentoring meetings can be negotiated and tested, with regular, frank follow-up discussions of their success and the need for further modification. The opportunity to seek and link to a more appropriate mentor must always be open.

Preventive measures might have avoided this sort of trouble. If the initial negotiation of the mentorship spelled out the responsibilities of both parties, negotiated a schedule of further meetings well in advance, provided

---

* We believe that it is better for a mentor to say "no" to a potential mentee than to agree to provide mentorship and then not be able to meet this commitment. We know it is tough to say "no" to a potential mentee, especially one who is really struggling, but taking on too many mentees isn't fair to any of them.

time-saving alternatives to face-to-face sessions (via telephone, Skype, or Twitter), allowed meetings on common issues with all a mentor's mentees in attendance, stated the absolute need to show up for meetings, and pre-scheduled periodic evaluations of how well these meetings are serving the mentoring functions and how their structure and function could be improved, this mess might have been prevented. If the initial terms of reference didn't do this at the start, now's the time to pull them out, spell out the responsibilities of each party to the relationship, and prevent these issues arising again in the future.

Mentoring meetings stop happening

A diagnosis is required, and one of the pair should track down the other and insist on a meeting to find out why. Since it is unlikely that the mentee has outgrown their need for at least some sort of mentoring (Dave Sackett is still getting mentored 53 years after his medical graduation), they should not be allowed to fall by the wayside. On the one hand, they may already have acquired another mentor, better suited to their interests, aspirations, needs, and style, which is a cause for celebration and closure of the original mentorship. On the other hand, through differences of interests, aspirations, needs, and style between the original mentor and mentee, they have simply drifted apart and the mentee needs to be offered a new and more attuned mentor. Once again, the generation, at the outset, of a schedule for regular meetings well in advance, when not fulfilled, would have achieved the early diagnosis of this failing mentorship and would have prevented the mentee from a prolonged period with not-active mentoring. In addition, those mentoring programs that require recertification of every mentorship every year (e.g. by requiring annual reports signed by both parties) will diagnose this failure.

The second cluster of mentorships in trouble arises from abuses of power. Because mentors wield so much power in determining the success or failure of their mentees, and because mentees (especially junior faculty and trainees) possess so little power to counteract abuse, credible mentoring programs include clear avenues of redress, including ombudsmen to whom mentees can come in confidence.

Failure to complete agreed-upon tasks

Again excepting the rare emergency, the repeated failure by either the mentor or mentee to do what they pledged to do at the end of the previous meeting is a symptom of a mentorship (or one of its members) in trouble. The diagnosis and prognosis are graver when the culprit is the mentor (with their far greater experience in knowing how much they can prepare, how quickly) and may call for euthanasia (of the link, that is) and transfer to a new mentor.

When mentees are at fault, our surveyed colleagues' responses ranged from sweet reason through tough love to asking the mentee to find another mentor. But all began with a frank discussion of what wasn't getting done by mentees, and why. This probe may reveal several treatable causes. New mentees often agree to tasks that are doable but too large for them to finish by an agreed date; however, if paring down† their assignment fails to meet with success, a further search for the diagnosis is required. Similarly, mentees may discover that they don't understand (or cannot apply) the methods required for completing an agreed task; as before, if this is a recurring problem and they're falling behind in their mastery of basic methodology, a deeper diagnosis must be sought.

The most frustrating and perplexing (for mentors) and prognostically ominous (for mentees) failures occur when mentees fail to meet agreed-upon deadlines for delivering drafts of theses or manuscripts for publication (especially when there are no intervening emergencies, prior warnings, or cries for help). Emergency, accurate diagnosis is essential, because if this pattern persists the mentee cannot succeed in an academic setting in which their promotion and tenure is largely dependent upon timely refereed publications in high-impact journals.

Easily remediable causes include:
- simple lack of experience in organizing, outlining and writing about anything
- lack of experience writing about scientific methods and results
- lack of experience writing about this particular subject matter.

Moreover, these causes should have been detected and treated back at the initiation of the mentorship through duplicate-blind reviews of research grants and manuscripts, and assigning small, doable writing tasks as routine assignments for regular mentoring sessions.‡

A less easy, but often remediable cause is "situational writing anxiety", in which taking on the specific writing task provokes so much apprehension and pessimism (not manifested in carrying out other tasks such as teaching or patient care) that its victim is simply unable to put words onto paper [1]. Again, however, this should have been detected much earlier and "desensitized" by providing and discussing plenty of examples of the required organization and composition and helping mentees compose just sentences, then paragraphs, then complete documents [2].

---

† Mentors can try to cut the task into smaller, stepped components and establish a modified timeline for each so that the task doesn't seem overwhelming to the mentee.

‡ One of our colleagues asks potential mentees to provide a two-page summary of their academic goals and plans to complete these goals before he agrees to provide mentorship; he uses this strategy to assess their writing skills.

Mentees with dysgraphia will almost certainly have identified themselves early on, and may already be utilizing strategies and tactics to assist their writing. Negotiating their outputs can take this into account.

That leaves the inexplicable failure of some mentees to meet deadlines. Mentors faced with this situation should, with the consent of their mentee, consult widely with their colleagues in an effort to identify and overcome the cause for this otherwise academically-fatal disorder.

Trouble from abuses of power

The second cluster of mentorships in trouble arises from abuses of power. Because mentors wield so much power in determining the success or failure of their mentees, and because mentees (especially junior faculty and trainees) possess so little power to counteract abuse, credible mentoring programs include clear avenues of redress, including ombudsmen to whom mentees can come in confidence.

Subversion of a mentee's interests to serve those of their mentor

Mentees gain valuable new skills and knowledge by taking on sub-projects of their mentor's research, or by writing an occasional report or commentary about their mentor's work, both conducted under their guidance. Moreover, mentees often seek to work with specific mentors because they share specific subject-matter interests and wish to work on the same family of research questions. An occasional mentor, however, regards mentees as research assistants, ignores their interests and aspirations, and exploits them as free hands to pursue only the mentor's interests. This stifling of the mentee's other interests stunts their growth and imperils their careers, and the resulting disillusion risks turning them off of academic pursuits altogether. Although mentees in these intolerable situations have occasionally come to the authors for help, this hit-and-miss system misses some exploited mentees, and a mentoring program worthy of the name provides clear lines of redress[§] and easy, confidential access to an ombudsman.

Theft of lead authorship

Occasionally we have become involved in cases in which mentees have done the lion's share of the work in designing, executing, analyzing, and writing up a project, only to discover that their mentors insist on lead authorship of the resulting publication. The damage to the mentee is twofold here: they

---

[§] Some mentorship programs have "mentorship facilitators" within each clinical division, who serve this purpose.

are not only robbed of recognition for this specific piece of work, but also robbed of a positive ethos in which academics support one another and respect each other's "ownership" of ideas and bodies of work. The former damage can be reversed by appeal to senior authority, ideally through an ombudsman, but the latter disillusion often impairs mentees' subsequent interactions with colleagues over the free exchange of ideas, and lessens their career satisfaction. The mentee should be assisted in linking to a new mentor. The offending mentor should be at least reprimanded, if not disbarred from future mentoring. For the prevention of both harms, the initiation of a mentee's research project should include preparing and filing a document that lists the order of authorship of reports arising from it. During the initial mentorship meeting, intellectual property should be discussed and this should be reiterated whenever a new project or manuscript idea is explored.

Theft of ideas

Worse yet is the case in which a mentee has generated a truly original research idea that has not previously occurred to their mentor, only to find that their mentor has presented that idea as their own in presentations, publications, and grant applications. Again, access to an ombudsman is vital in such cases, and if a dispute over ownership ensues, a formal investigation is required to sort it out. If theft is proven, a new mentor should be immediately provided and the guilty mentor should face condign punishment and be banned from future mentoring.

Bullying

The repeated, aggressive behavior by a mentor that is intended to hurt their mentee, emotionally or even physically is, quite simply, intolerable. Again, easy access to both an ombudsman and appropriate counseling and health services is essential in any program. If bullying is confirmed, a new mentor should be immediately provided and the guilty mentor should face condign punishment and be banned from future mentoring.

Sexual harassment

When mentors subject their mentees to intimidation, bullying or coercion of a sexual nature, or promise academic rewards in exchange for sexual favors, their behavior is not only intolerable; in most jurisdictions it is illegal. As before, easy access to both an ombudsman and appropriate counseling and health services is essential in any program. And, as before, if sexual harassment is established a new mentor should be immediately provided and the guilty mentor not only banned from future mentoring but reported to the police.

Trouble from true love on an unequal footing

True love

To close on a happier note (but, nonetheless, one that requires intervention), most of us know of situations in which relations between mentors and mentees evolve into mutually respectful, supportive, and non-exploitative love that may last for decades. While the phenomenon is not subject to intervention, the mentorship is. Because of the power difference between mentor and mentee, continuing the mentorship can harm both parties. If the couple doesn't recognize this early on and arrange for another mentor to take over those responsibilities, their friends and superiors should make sure that this occurs. Similarly, if the mentor and mentee become great friends, it may become more challenging to continue the traditional mentor–mentee relationship and the mentee should be linked to other mentors. The initial relationship often evolves into "peer mentorship."

Bottom line and scenario resolutions:

1 *The repeated unexplained no-shows at scheduled mentorship meetings by two mentees and two mentors.* You interview them individually. One of the mentees reluctantly comes to your office, appears severely depressed, and admits suicidal plans; you arrange immediate inpatient care and educate their shaken mentor on the recognition and management of depression. The second mentee states their mentor "is a nice guy" but not at all equipped to deal with their emerging field of research interest; after a brief discussion with the mentorship coordinator, you challenge the mentee to discuss this misalignment with their mentor; they do so, and both agree to reassignments. The first mentor in question angrily states that he's far too busy to "baby-sit" first-year graduate students; you discuss him with the mentorship coordinator, who relieves him (possibly to be considered mentoring of more senior colleagues at a later date) and helps the mentee link with a suitable mentor. The second mentor in question reveals to you that he is undergoing some personal family issues that have impacted his availability to meet with mentors and together you decide to find alternate mentors for his mentees until his situation is more settled.

2 *The repeated failure of a mentee to complete agreed tasks between sessions.* At interview, the quite bright mentee reluctantly reports moderately severe dyslexia and severe dysgraphia (undiscovered during their admission to the program), which renders them incapable of writing more than a few words at a sitting. After discussion with the mentorship coordinator, the mentee is offered alternative reporting methods and provided ongoing educational supports. The mentee flourishes.

3 *The case in which mentoring meetings have simply stopped happening.* You interview the mentee and discover that they have lost interest in a research

career, have stopped going to classes, and have been accepted into a medical sub-specialty training program for the coming year. You inform the mentorship coordinator, who chides the mentee for not having discussed their changing situation with their mentor, and chides the mentor for not having pursued a diagnosis for the cessation.

4 *The complaint from a mentee that his research interests have been subverted to serve those of his mentor.* The mentor in question is an aggressive, world-renowned researcher whose mentees usually bend to his will, gladly accept his ideas for their research, get effectively mentored within his content and methodological areas, and become highly successful academics. After discussion with the mentorship coordinator, a "no-fault" divorce is arranged and the mentee flourishes with a new, "non-directive" mentor.

5 *The charge from a mentee that her mentor insisted on lead authorship on a paper describing research into her original idea and in which she had done most of the work.* After determining that there was no prior, written agreement about authorship at the start of the project, you and the mentorship coordinator hand over to the department chair, who investigates, confirms the charge, and restores the mentee to lead authorship. Although profoundly grateful for being rescued and linked to another mentor, the mentee professes a growing distrust of senior academics and ultimately pursues an entirely clinical career in a different city.

6 *The charge from a mentee that his mentor stole his research idea.* You inform the mentorship coordinator, who immediately (but confidentially) refers the charge to the department chair. The department chair immediately contacts the mentor.

7 *The complaint from a mentee that they are being bullied by their mentor.* You interview the mentee, document their charge, educate them about your university's bullying policy and procedures, immediately connect them to that service, and inform the mentorship coordinator.

8 *The charge from a mentee that she has been sexually harassed by her mentor.* You immediately arrange a "safe place" for the mentee, cancel the mentorship, call in your university's sexual harassment team and ombudsperson, and inform the mentorship coordinator.

9 *A concern from a mentor that her mentee does not respond to her feed-back or suggestions.* You discuss this concern with the mentor who tells you that the mentee has had several bad experiences with previous "tor-mentors" who bullied him and he perceived that they stole his intellectual property. The mentor feels that this is impacting the mentee's ability to trust anyone, including her. You also discuss this with the mentee who confirms this and you encourage both of them to attend a workshop on communication for mentors and mentees; you check in with them in three months. At the follow-up meetings, you determine that additional support is required for the mentee and you refer them to a psychologist for additional emotional support.

10 *The rumor that one of your mentor–mentee dyads are living together.* You gently and confidentially confront the mentor and, if the rumor is confirmed, ask the mentorship coordinator to dissolve the mentorship and reassign its members.

Note that many of these situations require the mentor or the mentorship coordinator to do some digging; on the surface these issues may be perceived to be bad behavior on the part of the mentor or mentee but additional data gathering is required to make an accurate diagnosis of the problem and target appropriate interventions.

References

1. The Writing Center. Writing anxiety. Available at: http://writingcenter.unc.edu /handouts/writing-anxiety/. Accessed December 2012.
2. The Writing Center. Handouts. Available at: http://writingcenter.unc.edu /handouts/. Accessed December 2012.

Chapter 6 How can you initiate and maintain a mentorship progam?

Scenario

At the end of your first year as an academic clinician-investigator in a big, busy clinical department, (200 faculty members, 10 clinical divisions) you've just finished discussing your annual review with your department chair. She tells you that you're doing extremely well for a new faculty member, which is a great relief to you. Although you think you've done pretty well (in the past year, you received a peer-reviewed development grant, first-authored two papers and co-authored four others, have a systematic review in press, have an abstract accepted for a national meeting, are enjoying your time on the clinical service, and the medical students and residents submitted glowing assessments of your bedside teaching), you feel pressed for time, worry about your work–life balance, and wonder whether you're "on the right track" for a successful and enjoyable academic career. Although you've received encouragement from several senior members of the department, you've been conscious of how busy they are and don't want to impose on their jam-packed schedules to ask for advice. But now, stimulated by a recent workshop on mentorship that you attended at an academic meeting and emboldened by your chair's praise, you tell her that you and some of your colleagues are concerned about the lack of a formal mentorship program in the department. The department chair challenged you to review the evidence on mentorship and to make a case for it. You presented this to her (see Chapter 1) and based on your successful pitch to her, she's now asked you to develop a mentorship program.

You'll recognize the above scenario from the start and end of Chapter 1. Here in Chapter 6, we'll address how to plan and implement a mentorship program. In Chapter 7, we'll outline how to evaluate and sustain the program in your institution.

In describing an approach to planning and implementing a mentorship program, we'll draw on three systematic reviews (moderate-quality evidence)

Mentorship in Academic Medicine, First Edition. Sharon E. Straus and David L. Sackett.
© 2014 John Wiley & Sons, Ltd. Published 2014 by John Wiley & Sons, Ltd.

of mentorship [1–3], updated by newer searches to identify any more recent articles. This update identified an additional four relevant studies (two surveys [4, 5], one validation study of a tool to measure the impact of mentorship [6], and one qualitative study [7]) that focused on the development of a faculty mentorship program. As before, we didn't find any randomized trials comparing different mentorship programs or different education programs for mentors and mentees.

Our approach to implementing mentorship programs is also informed by the Knowledge to Action Framework [8] derived from a review of more than 30 theories of planned action. In this model (Figure 6.1), the "central knowledge creation funnel" represents knowledge generation and synthesis, in this case the knowledge in support of mentorship that was described in Chapter 1. The "action" parts of the cycle are based on "planned action"

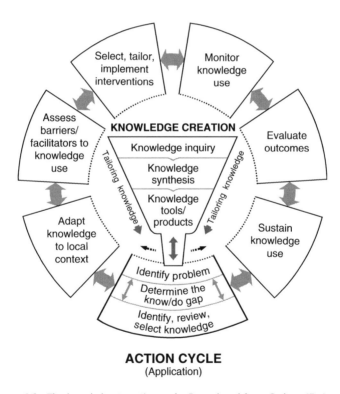

ACTION CYCLE
(Application)

Figure 6.1 The knowledge to action cycle. Reproduced from Graham ID, Logan J, Harrison MB, Straus SE, Tetroe J, Caswell W, Robinson N. Lost in knowledge translation: time for a map? J Contin Educ Health Prof. 2006;26(1):13–24, with permission from John Wiley and sons.

theories of how to engineer change in health care systems and groups. Included in this action cycle are identifying the problem or completing a needs assessment; assessing the determinants of knowledge use; selecting, tailoring and implementing an intervention; and determining strategies for ensuring sustained knowledge use. We have found this approach helpful when developing mentorship programs [9].

How do you assess the need for mentorship in your department?

Once you have decided (based on the evidence presented in Chapter 1) that mentoring does more good than harm, the next step is to find out what your department needs in order to provide it to those who will benefit from receiving it, especially during the early stages of their academic development. To succeed in this next step, you need the "right" people, using the "right" tools to identify and quantify these needs. We suggest that the right people comprise a "stakeholder advisory group" that includes faculty from the relevant career paths (e.g. clinician-educators*/researchers/administrators) and ranks (e.g. junior, mid-career, and senior faculty), and relevant academic administrators (e.g. division director, department chairs, and others). Invited faculty should include those already acknowledged to be excellent mentors (e.g. recipients of mentoring or teaching awards) and those expressing keen support for the proposal (who could function as local champions). Finally, to this group you add a secretariat to document what they do and a support staff to apply the right tools for assessing needs.

This needs assessment should follow a systematic process for determining both the size and the nature of the gap between the current and a more desirable mentoring program [10]. This gap can usefully be described in terms of what your target groups say that they need (so-called "felt needs"), how they already are acting to fulfill them (so-called "expressed needs"), what a bunch of experts like us suggest they really need (so-called "normative" needs), and how their needs compare to other groups at other institutions (so-called "comparative" needs) [10].

The assessment for felt and expressed needs can usefully identify needs at both the organizational and individual level and can take many forms

---

* In our review of the literature (as discussed in Chapter 1) we found that clinician-educators are much less likely to have mentors than clinician-scientists and take longer to achieve promotion, although it's not clear if these two facts are causally related. Nonetheless, this evidence demands that special attention be paid to neglected groups (in this case, educators) when developing mentorship programs.

including reviews of documents, surveys, interviews, and focus groups amongst relevant individuals. For example, a needs assessment at the institution level might include surveys of all faculty (e.g. to determine how many have or want a mentor), surveys of administrators (e.g. to determine their perceptions of the need for mentorship), reviews of faculty annual reports and CVs (to assess productivity and mentee supervision), and a review of institutional criteria for promotion and tenure (e.g. to determine whether mentorship is valued in decisions on promotion and tenure). At the individual level, a needs assessment can similarly include a survey (e.g. to explore academic self-efficacy, satisfaction with mentors), focus groups or interviews (e.g. to explore the quality of the mentoring relationship), or assessment of CVs and annual activity reports (to assess time to promotion and productivity). Surveys of faculty members can also be used to understand readiness to be a mentor or mentee and scholarly interests; this data can then be used later as a mentor database for mentees to review when trying to find a mentor.

There are no tools for assessing mentorship needs (felt, expressed, normative, or comparative needs) that have been assessed for accuracy in the peer-reviewed literature but we found two papers describing potential tools [4, 11]. Mitch Feldman and colleagues developed and implemented a survey across faculty members at all four professional schools at University of California, San Francisco (UCSF) to elicit their perceptions of and needs for mentorship [4]. This instrument included questions on demographics, current mentoring relationships (including topics discussed with mentors, identification of mentors, and challenges with mentorship) and academic self-efficacy. Their definition and assessment of academic self-efficacy included rating of academic skills such as identification of professional goals and interests and identification of requirements for advancement and promotion at UCSF [4]. Faculty dissatisfaction with mentoring that was identified in this survey stimulated the creation of a cross-faculty mentorship program at UCSF. Our search of the grey literature identified other tools developed for both assessing the need for mentorship and for creating a mentor database. For example, the Faculty of Medicine at the University of Ottawa in Canada developed a form for potential mentors and mentees that asks them to rate their competencies in certain areas such as research and writing manuscripts [12]. However, there are no data on the impact of this tool on successful mentorship. When selecting a tool for needs assessment, we suggest that readers generate and vigorously pre-test a brief, user-friendly questionnaire that balances the need for information against the limited time that their target faculty and trainees have available for (or are willing to devote to) completing surveys. And, given the abundant evidence that those who immediately complete and return surveys provide different opinions from those who return them late or not at all, the follow-up of non-responders should be vigorous pursued until the overall return rate exceeds 80%.

How do you assess the barriers and facilitators to implementation of a mentorship program?

In this next step, you identify the factors that impede (barriers) and promote (facilitators) the implementation of your mentorship program. You can supplement the results of the survey with evidence from the literature. For example, the barriers to mentorship that we described in Chapter 2 occurred both at the individual (mentor and mentee) and institutional levels [3]. At the individual mentor level they include lack of time, lack of academic credit for mentorship, lack of experience, and lack of confidence in their mentoring ability [3, 13, 14]. At the individual mentee level they include lack of time, lack of availability of mentors with similar scholarly interests, and lack of experience as a mentee.[†] At the level of institutions, barriers include a lack of recognition of the importance of mentoring, an absence of training opportunities for mentoring and of mentors, and a lack of resources to support mentoring programs [3, 13, 14].

This latter evidence can be used to generate the issues to address in surveys, interviews, and focus groups. The responses will identify the most significant barriers and facilitators to implementation at your institution (this is often described in the implementation and education literature as "contextualizing" the intervention to the local setting) so that you can develop strategies to overcome the barriers and exploit the facilitators.

How do you develop and implement the mentorship program?

The results of your needs assessments and the identification of your local barriers and facilitators will form the basis for the 'nuts-and-bolts' design and development of your local mentorship program.

1 Use the needs and barriers assessments to identify your local opinion leaders (or "mentorship champions") to publicly advocate for your program, identify current and potential mentors, and support their development

---

[†] As outlined in Chapter 1, we found in our literature review that lack of mentors seems to be a particular problem for small institutions, institutions with scholarly interests in very few fields, clinician educators, and senior faculty members.

within their divisions [9]. Although a "mentorship champion" might be a department chair or division head, this confounds advocacy with control of resources, and it will be difficult to determine whether volunteer mentors are responding to the former or the latter inducement. These champions can also develop and employ strategies to detect and rescue or, if necessary, dissolve mentorships in trouble (see Chapter 5).

2 Design and hold highly interactive, small-group workshops to address issues such as deciding whether to become a mentor, understanding the characteristics of effective mentors and mentees, matching mentors and mentees, running mentorship meetings, optimizing communication between mentees and their mentors, developing strategies and tactics for tracking mentees' career progress, and other topics nominated by your target audiences (which should include mentors and mentees).

3 Create or copy more formal mentor-training courses, or sponsor prospective mentors to courses held elsewhere. And, consider providing them with resources to develop a similar workshop at your institution.

4 Create (or reproduce) both printed and online education materials for mentors and mentees, including mentorship checklists, contracts for mentees, individual development plans, and progress reports (such as those we've provided in this book and on the accompanying website).

5 Create hassle-free systems for documenting and evaluating mentoring successes.

6 Lobby deans and other mandarins to have mentoring count greatly in promotion and tenure; this should involve including mentorship on annual activity reports and academic CVs.

7 Create other institutional strategies for celebrating and awarding successful mentorship.[‡]

8 Promote this culture change by requiring prospective faculty to discuss mentorship as part of their recruitment process.

Based on the available evidence, we suggest that mentorship programs have multiple components (including some of the elements described in the list above) and be formalized, with assistance provided for identification of mentors [3]. A mentor should be offered to every faculty member, regardless of their career path (e.g. clinician, clinician teacher/educator, clinician investigator/scientist, clinician administrator) and stage, recognizing that the needs of junior faculty clearly are different from those of their senior colleagues, and that clinician-educators may want and need different mentoring than

---

[‡] When chairs and deans tell Dave Sackett how important mentors are for the success of their institutions, he asks them why – in view of this – their "best" mentors aren't offered reserved (or at least free) parking.

clinician-investigators. Indeed, as discussed in Chapter 1, more advanced colleagues' mentoring needs are often ignored within institutions, despite their being more likely to be considering significant changes to their career paths, taking on new leadership roles, or transitioning to retirement.

When resources are scarce, it makes sense to start by mentoring junior faculty and then extending the process to more senior colleagues over time (where peer-mentoring begins to take over). In addition, as mentioned in Chapter 3, team mentorship or mentorship at a distance could be considered to meet the needs of the individual mentee, accompanied by funding to support annual in-person meetings between distance-mentors and mentees [13].

While descriptions of use of mentorship contracts (outlining the responsibility and accountability for the relationship and signed by the mentor and mentee) exist, their benefits aren't clear (low-quality evidence) [1, 3]. Progress reports by the mentor and mentee can be useful to promote accountability but their contents should be kept confidential. Divisions or departments can ask for a few items to be included on the annual activity report required by faculty members, such as have they met with their mentor over the last year, and can they comment on the quality of the relationship with the mentor. They can also ask that the mentor review the faculty member's annual activity report including short- and long-term goals and to sign off on this before it's submitted to the department chair. However, we strongly caution against making the mentorship process overly bureaucratic as each form that needs to be completed means another obstacle to effective mentorship and can turn people off; we'd all rather have people spend their time doing mentorship than documenting it!

There are several mentorship programs currently documented at academic institutions, and the URLs for some of them appear at the end of this chapter (and will be kept up to date on our website: www.mentorshipacademic medicine.com). The mentorship program created by Mitch Feldman at UCSF deserves special attention: it targets junior faculty (up to associate professor) across four professional faculties (medicine, nursing, pharmacy, and dentistry) [4], includes mentorship facilitators within each department or division, has implemented education sessions for both mentors and mentees, and has instituted annual awards for achievement in mentoring. Gratifyingly, a 2010 survey of UCSF faculty found increased satisfaction with both the availability and quality of mentoring since the initiation of their mentoring program [16].

Moreover, as part of an NIH-funded Clinical and Translational Science Institute, this same group developed a mentorship development program to train mid-career and early senior clinical and translational research faculty in the art and science of mentoring [5, 17]. It employs case-based seminars that focus on not only the strategies and tactics of effective mentoring, but also provide instrumental (i.e. "nuts and bolts") and psychosocial support for mentors. Evaluated in a before/after survey of 26 participants who completed this course, supplemented by up to 3 years of follow-up among 38 graduates, most felt it had an impact on their mentorship skills and increased their confidence in mentoring (no data are yet available on recruitment, retention, or career productivity). This program also hosts a website with additional resources and tools to support mentorship, such as an individual development plan [5]. A similar mentorship development program has been launched at the Cleveland Clinic although there is no evaluation to date [18]. We will provide updates on these programs on this book's website.

Once established, energies go to evolving, improving, and sustaining it, and this requires monitoring the mentorship program and its impact. We'll take these challenges up in Chapter 7.

Gaps in research

Most of the evidence on development of mentorship programs is descriptive and there is little quantitative data to guide our efforts. For example, it would be useful to have precise and accurate tools to assess the need for mentorship, knowledge about optimal strategies for implementing a mentorship program, and how to adapt them to different settings. This provides an excellent opportunity for institutions interested in mentorship to work together to design and carry out multi-site evaluations of mentorship programs. Inclusion of qualitative elements in this evaluation would improve our understanding of the "active ingredients" (i.e. most effective components) of all our mentorship programs.

Bottom line and scenario resolution

You form an advisory group with representation from faculty across the clinical divisions within your department, career paths, and ranks. Together, you create a needs assessment (see Box 6.1) including a list of barriers to mentorship, and ask respondents to rate the significance of each using a Likert scale rating from 1 to 5. Your group sent the survey via email to all department members with an introduction from the department chair. Email reminders to complete the survey were sent one and two weeks after the initial email, and further email and phone calls persisted until the response rate achieved 88%.

Your group uses the results of the survey to design interviews with faculty members, and your research associate conducted 20 of them, including faculty from every career path and rank. Your group used the results from the survey and interviews to design and launch a mentorship program with the following components:

1 Creation of a policy that clearly states the mandate for mentorship[$] and sets down the guidelines for its development and implementation (with endorsement by the department chair).

2 Identification of a mentorship facilitator in each division. For each division in the department, this person was identified in the survey and confirmed following interviews and discussions with the department chair. Each facilitator will serve as a mentorship champion in their division and will facilitate linkage between mentors and mentees, provide access to resources to support mentorship such as a mentorship toolkit, encourage enrollment and attendance at departmental workshops on mentorship, and function as a mediator for mentorships in trouble. After some wrangling, your department chair agreed to 0.2 FTE salary supplementation for each facilitator, plus a part-time assistant.

3 Requirement that each new and junior faculty member in the department identify a mentor within the first year of the program, and commit to meet this person regularly and, in particular, within two months of their annual academic appointment review (your department chair holds annual academic appointment reviews with each member).

4 Development of a presentation on the mentorship program by the department chair and one member of your advisory group that will be included in the annual orientation meeting for new faculty that is held by your department each fall.

5 Creation of a core group of mentorship resources for use across all divisions in your department, including:

   a) A workshop for 'mentorship facilitators' to teach them their role and an array of strategies for facilitating linkage of mentors and mentees. Strategies include access to a mentor database and the use of departmental and divisional meetings or informal social gatherings for "speed mentoring". Your department chair worked with division directors to provide $1500 for networking activities within each division.

   b) A workshop for mentors and mentees including discussion of roles and responsibilities of each and communication strategies.

   c) Printed and web-based educational materials for mentors and mentees, including the mentorship meeting checklist that appears in Chapter 4, mentorship guidelines, the revised annual activity report and revised academic CV (with its documentation of mentorship, including number of mentees, and outcomes of mentorship such as receiving grants, awards, and publications). The revised annual activity report (this report is required for completion by each division member and is reviewed by the division director and department chair) also includes a section to indicate that the document has been reviewed and discussed by the mentor and mentee.

[$]We have included a number of links to sample policy documents on the website that accompanies this book (www.mentorshipacademicmedicine.com) and encourage readers to review these rather than create one from scratch!

d) Mentorship "stories", providing exemplars of both effective mentorships and "mentorships in trouble".
6 Rewarding mentorship in promotion and tenure.
7 Creating mentorship awards, nominated by mentees.

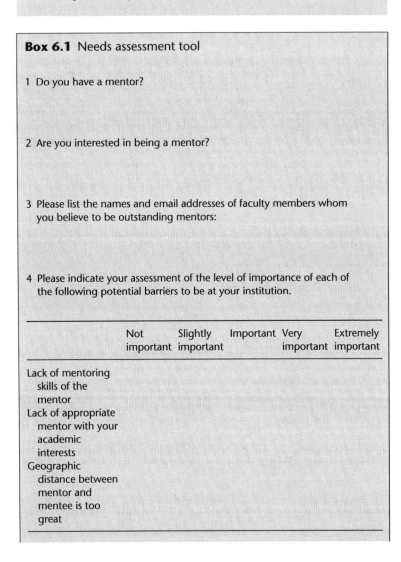

Box 6.1 Needs assessment tool

1 Do you have a mentor?

2 Are you interested in being a mentor?

3 Please list the names and email addresses of faculty members whom
  you believe to be outstanding mentors:

4 Please indicate your assessment of the level of importance of each of
  the following potential barriers to be at your institution.

	Not important	Slightly important	Important	Very important	Extremely important
Lack of mentoring skills of the mentor					
Lack of appropriate mentor with your academic interests					
Geographic distance between mentor and mentee is too great					

	Not important	Slightly important	Important	Very important	Extremely important
Lack of appropriate mentor of same gender					
Lack of appropriate mentor of same race/culture					
Mentor takes advantages of mentee					
Mentor steals idea for grants and/or publication from mentee					
Mentor competes with mentee for resources					
Mentor doesn't have sufficient time to meet with mentee					
Mentee doesn't have sufficient time to meet with mentor					
Mentor sexually harassing mentee					
Mentor verbally abusing mentee					
Mentor directs activities of mentee					
Lack of academic recognition for mentors					
Lack of financial incentive for mentors					
Lack of inclusion of mentorship in promotion criteria					

5 If you have answered yes to Question 1, do you believe your mentor has played a role in your career development and success? Please indicate your level of agreement with the following statements.

	Strongly disagree	Disagree	Neither agree nor disagree	Agree	Strongly Agree
a) My mentor had a negative impact on my career development					
b) My mentor had a negative impact on my career success					
c) My mentor had a positive impact on my career success					
d) My mentor had a positive impact on my career development					
e) My mentor and I meet regularly to discuss my progress					
f) My mentor helped me to be strategic about research opportunities					
g) My mentor helped me to be strategic about grant opportunities					
h) My mentor helped me to be strategic about presenting my research at academic meetings					

References

1. Sambunjak D, Straus SE, Marusic A. Mentoring in academic medicine: a systematic review. JAMA 2006; 296; 1103–15.
2. Straus SE, Straus C, Tzanetos K. Career choice in academic medicine: a systematic review. J Gen Int Med 2006; 21: 1222–9.
3. Sambunjak D, Straus SE, Marusic A. A systematic review of qualitative research of the meaning and characteristics of mentoring in academic medicine. J Gen Int Med 2010; 25: 72–8.

4. Feldman MD, Arean PA, Marshall SJ, et al. Does mentoring matter? Med Ed Online 2010; 15: 5063.
5. Feldman MD, et al. Training the next generation of research mentors. Clin Trans Sci 2009; 2: 216–21.
6. Dilmore TC, Rubio DM, Cohen E, et al. Psychometric properties of the Mentor Role Instrument when used in the academic medicine setting. Clin Trans Sci 2010; 3: 104–8.
7. Gusic ME, Zenni EA, Ludwig S, First LS. Strategies to design an effective mentorship program. J Ped 2009; 11: 173–4.
8. Graham ID, Logan J, Harrison MB, et al. Lost in knowledge translation: time for a map? J Cont Educ Health Prof 2006; 26: 13–24.
9. Straus SE, Graham I, Wong A, et al. Development of a mentorship strategy: A knowledge translation case study. J Cont Educ Health Prof 2008, 28: 117–22.
10. Lockyer J. Needs assessment: lessons learned. J Cont Educ Health Prof 1998; 18: 190–2.
11. Keyser DJ, Ladoski JM, Lara-Cinisomo S, et al. Advancing institutional efforts to support research mentorship. Acad Med 2008; 83: 217–25.
12. Mentorship assessment tool. Available at: http://www.medicine.uottawa.ca/genderequity/eng/mentoring.html. Accessed 25 May 2012.
13. Straus SE, Chatur F, Taylor M. Issues in the mentor-mentee relationship in academic medicine: qualitative study. Acad Med. 2009; 84: 135–9.
14. Straus SE, Johnson MO, Marquez C, Feldman MD. Characteristics of successful and failed mentoring relationships: qualitative study across two institutions. Acad Med 2013; 88: 82–9.
15. Johnson MO, Subak LL, Brown JS, et al. An innovative program to train health services researchers to be effective clinical and translational research mentors. Acad Med 2010; 85: 484–9.
16. UCSF Faculty Climate Survey, Executive Summary. Available at: http://academicaffairs.ucsf.edu/FacultyClimateSurvey/index.php. Accessed 21 August 2012.
17. Feldman MD, Steinauer J, Khalili M, et al. A mentorship development program for clinical translational scientists faculty leads to sustained, improved confidence in mentoring skills. Clin Transl Sci 2011; doi: 10.1111/j.1752-8062.2012.00419.
18. Blixen CE, Papp KK, Hull A, et al. Developing a mentorship program for clinician researchers. J Cont Educ Health Prof 2007; 27: 86–93.

For additional information on mentorship programs developed by various organizations and institutions, we have provided a list of URLs below and on the website that accompanies this book (accessed December 2012).

http://www.americanheart.org/presenter.jhtml?identifier=3016094
http://www.medschool.vcu.edu/ofid/facdev/facultymentoring.html
http://www.uwosh.edu/mentoring/faculty/
http://www.umassmed.edu/facultyadmin/mentoring/index.aspx
http://gumc.georgetown.edu/evp/facultyaffairs/mentoringprogram/usefullinksonmentorships/46720.html

http://www.schulich.uwo.ca/humanresources/facultymentorship/files/Admin
  /MentorshipProgram.pdf
http://deptmedicine.arizona.edu/faculty_mentoring/getting-started
http://www.medicine.uottawa.ca/genderequity/eng/mentoring.html
http://www.medicine.uottawa.ca/genderequity/eng/mentoring.html
http://academicaffairs.ucsf.edu/mentoring/

Chapter 7 **How can you evaluate the impact of a mentorship program?**

Scenario

It's been two years since your team launched the mentorship program for your department. All new faculty members (and a growing number of mid-career faculty) have mentors, are meeting regularly, and the departmental consensus is that it's a success (with only a couple of "mentorships in trouble", which were quickly diagnosed and treated). Indeed, responding to clamor from their disaffected junior faculty, three other departments have come to yours to find out how they might set up similar programs.

During your annual review with your chair, she asks if there's any "hard"' evidence that the mentorship program is making a difference. She wants you to prepare a report for the departmental retreat that will be held in three months; she says she'll use the information to decide whether to continue to fund the program. What would you like to have up your sleeve that you could pull out and hand to her in response to her question?

In describing an approach to evaluating a mentorship program in this chapter, we'll draw on our comprehensive literature review based on three systematic reviews (moderate-quality evidence) of mentorship [1–3], updated by newer searches to identify any more recent articles. When assessing mentorship programs, most authors of the studies we identified used surveys that they developed for their own studies (reporting on outcomes such as satisfaction with mentorship that was measured using a Likert scale) [1–3]. Some studies reported research productivity measured by peer-reviewed grant success and publications [4, 5]. From the updated search, we identified three studies describing validated tools for measuring impact of mentorship [6–8], and a fourth study that identified mentor competencies [9].

As discussed in Chapter 6, our approach to implementing a mentorship program is informed by the Knowledge to Action Framework [10], which

Mentorship in Academic Medicine, First Edition. Sharon E. Straus and David L. Sackett.
© 2014 John Wiley & Sons, Ltd. Published 2014 by John Wiley & Sons, Ltd.

is a conceptual framework for evidence implementation, based on a review of more than 30 theories of planned action; we have found it to be helpful when both developing and evaluating a mentorship program [11].

How do you measure the impact of your mentorship program?

Identifying the goals of the mentorship program and potential strategies for their measurement

The initial issues to consider when setting up an evaluation strategy are the goals of your mentorship program (for the mentees, the mentors, and the institution) and how can you align your measurement approach with these goals. For example, is the goal to increase access to mentors? To increase grants and publications received by clinician scientists? To enhance job satisfaction for faculty? Or, to increase retention of faculty? Ideally, you should be trying to nurture and support productive, happy faculty so you may want to achieve all of these outcomes.

We'll refer to Table 7.1 for our discussion of selecting goals for mentorship programs. We created this table from three sources: first, we used material from the study by Gusic and colleagues [12] that used mentorship discussions at workshops held during meetings of the American Pediatric Academic Society to describe potential outcomes from mentorship programs, including job satisfaction, satisfaction with the program, career productivity, and faculty retention; second, we expanded this list based on our literature review; and third, we used the Donabedian framework for measuring quality of care to categorize them (Table 7.1) as structural, process or outcome measures [13]. For each of these measures, we have identified potential strategies for data collection.

Structural measures focus on organizational aspects of service provision, which includes provision of mentors and mentorship workshops for example. Process indicators focus on the elements of the delivery of mentorship, such as experience with mentorship and job satisfaction. Outcome indicators refer to the ultimate goal(s) of mentorship, such as academic productivity, promotion and tenure, and retention of faculty. These measures can apply to the institution or individual (including the mentor and the mentee).

At the institutional level, structural measures include the availability of mentors or of a mentorship workshop within an institution. To measure these outcomes you could collect data (via surveys of faculty members or review of their annual activity reports) on the number of faculty members who are interested in being mentors, the proportion of faculty members who have a mentor, and the number of mentorship workshops that are available across

Table 7.1 Goals of mentorship programs and how to measure their attainment

A. Institutions		
Institutional structures		
Goals	What to measure	How to measure it
Presence of a mentoring program	Is there one?	Departmental and mentoring program annual reports
Availability of mentor training	Numbers and contents of mentoring workshops	Surveys of faculty and trainees
Presence of an ombudsperson	Is there one?	Ombudsperson annual report
Institutional processes		
Goals	What to measure	How to measure it
Participation in mentoring	Numbers of mentors Numbers of faculty and trainees who have mentors	Departmental and mentoring program annual reports Surveys of faculty and trainees
Meeting unmet needs for mentoring	Numbers of faculty and trainees who don't have mentors but want one	Surveys of faculty and trainees
Participation in mentor training	Number of faculty members who participated in a mentorship training program Numbers of mentors in training	Mentoring program attendance logs and annual reports
Participation of ombudsman	Numbers, types, and dispositions of problems brought/not brought to them	Ombudsperson annual report Surveys of mentors and mentees
Rewards for mentoring	Rewarding mentoring in departmental and institutional criteria for promotion and tenure "Perks" and privileges for mentors	Review of departmental and institutional criteria for promotion and tenure. Surveys of mentors
Institutional outcomes		
Goals	What to measure	How to measure it
Retention and academic promotion of mentors	Numbers of mentors retained at 5 and 10 years Numbers of mentors promoted	Departmental annual reports
Recruitment of new faculty enhanced by presence of a mentoring program	Numbers and proportions of recruits stating the presence of a mentoring program was important in their decision to join	Surveys of faculty recruited since the mentoring program was established

(continues)

Table 7.1   (Continued)

Goals	What to measure	How to measure it
Recruitment and academic success of former mentees	Numbers and proportions of former mentees recruited here and elsewhere Grant support, publications, and academic promotions of former mentees	Surveys of former mentees and examination of their CVs
Recruitment of new trainees enhanced by presence of a mentoring program	Numbers and proportions of recruits stating the presence of a mentoring program was important in their decision to join	Surveys of trainees recruited since the mentoring program was established
Export of mentoring program to other institutions	Numbers of other institutions coming for help Numbers of faculty recruited elsewhere to establish mentoring programs	Departmental and institutional annual reports Surveys of faculty recruited to other institutions
B. MENTEES		
Individual mentee structures		
Goals	What to measure	How to measure it
Participation in an organized mentoring system	Were they able to pick their mentor? Did they get a "good" mentor? Was a "manual" or other guidance on being a mentee available? Was a system for changing mentors available? Was an ombudsperson available?	
Individual mentee processes		
Goals	What to measure	How to measure it
Participation in an effective mentoring system	Did the format and frequency of mentoring sessions meet their needs? Did mentoring include priority-setting, time-management, dys-opportunities, knowledge-generation, knowledge-dissemination, academic milestones, academic dossiers, protection from sharks, and recruitment to their next job? Did mentor (or a more appropriate designate) address personal issues? Was the mentor's response to urgent problems swift and helpful?	Mentee surveys and interviews

Table 7.1 (Continued)

Goals	What to measure	How to measure it
Feeling competent as a researcher, educator, (and clinician)	Self-efficacy with academic skills [9]	Mentee surveys and interviews
Feeling that they've "graduated" to a good academic job	Job-description Job-satisfaction	Mentee surveys and interviews

Individual mentee outcomes		
Goals	What to measure	How to measure it
Productivity	Peer-reviewed grants awarded Peer-reviewed publications	Mentee CVs
Promotion	Time-course of academic rank	
Work–life balance and avoidance of burn-out		Mentee CVs, surveys and interviews

C. MENTORS		
Individual mentor structures		
Goals	What to measure	How to measure it
Participation in an organized mentoring system	Was a mentor-training program available? Were they able to pick their mentees? Was a "manual" or other guidance on being a mentor available? Was a system for changing mentees available? Was an ombudsperson available?	Departmental and institutional documents

Individual mentor processes		
Goals	What to measure	How to measure it
Participation in an effective mentoring system	Were they able to limit their number of mentees? Was help available for mentee issues outside their expertise? Was help available when they couldn't help inadequately performing mentees?	Mentor surveys and interviews

(continues)

Table 7.1 (Continued)

Goals	What to measure	How to measure it
Feeling competent as a mentor Enjoying mentoring Feeling that their mentoring efforts have been appreciated by their mentees Pride in their mentees Feeling that mentoring has enhanced their academic career despite its time and energy commitments Feeling that their mentoring efforts have been appreciated by their institution	Mentor perceptions	Mentor surveys and interviews
Individual mentor outcomes		
Goals	What to measure	How to measure it
Productivity Promotion	Peer-reviewed grants awarded Peer-reviewed publications Academic progress	Mentor CVs

the institution. Process measures include participation in a mentorship workshop, which can be assessed using attendance logs for these events. Ultimately, mentorship programs are developed to impact outcomes such as recruitment and retention of faculty; this data can be collected using departmental annual reports.

At the individual level, several measures can be considered for assessing impact of mentorship on mentors or mentees. Structural measures include the time available to meet a mentor and the method of communication used by mentors and mentees (e.g. use of email or in-person meetings). This data could be collected using surveys of mentors and mentees. Process measures include items like self-efficacy in academic medicine, job satisfaction, experience with mentorship, and experience with the mentorship workshops.

We identified four studies that reported on various tools or frameworks for assessing process measures.

1 In a survey of faculty members, Feldman and colleagues used a validated scale (including six questions scored using a Likert scale from 1 = weak and 9 = strong agreement for confidence in key academic skills) to assess self-efficacy in academic medicine [8], and found faculty members with mentors had a higher self-efficacy score than those without a mentor

(mean score 6.1 [SD 1.4] versus 5.4 [SD 1.4], $p < 0.001$) [8]. It's unclear whether this result translated into improved productivity or retention of faculty.

2   Dutta and colleagues assessed the impact of mentorship in a survey of faculty members and used validated scales for job satisfaction and job-related well-being [6]. They found that mentorship was associated with increased job satisfaction and well-being.

3   We identified one validated tool for assessing mentoring roles at the individual level [7]. This tool was developed using Kram's theory of mentoring roles, and characterized mentoring relationships in terms of career and psychosocial development [7]. It includes 33 items: 15 items measure perceptions of 5 career roles (sponsor, coach, protector, challenger, promoter) and 18 items measure perceptions of 6 psychosocial roles (friend, social associate, parent, role model, counselor, acceptor) [7]. It was tested in 141 research trainees involved with a clinical and translational science institute at the University of Pittsburgh who were also asked to provide a general rating of their mentoring relationship and its effectiveness. The tool was found to have good reliability (Pearson correlation coefficients ≥ 0.60 for all items) and validity (concurrent validity, Pearson correlation coefficient > 0.55 for psychosocial and career roles and general ratings of mentorship) in capturing the nature of mentoring. Responsiveness of this tool to change in the mentorship relationship over time has not been assessed. Moreover, it has not been validated against measures such as mentee and mentor productivity or retention.

4   Abedin and colleagues completed a study to develop a framework for mentorship competencies [9]. They completed focus groups with scholars and mentors across four US sites and integrated this material with the results of a literature review, review of mentor evaluation forms, and discussion by an expert panel. They identified 19 competencies aligned across 6 themes for mentors for clinician scientists, including communication and relationship management, psychosocial support, career and professional development, professional enculturation and scientific integrity, resource development, and clinician-scientist development. While they provide definitions and examples of each of the competencies, it is not clear how to measure them and thus their validity has not been assessed. We mention this paper to highlight a target for future research for those interested in mentorship.

To capture additional information on individual experience with mentorship, qualitative data can be collected using interviews with mentors and mentees. Several studies have provided interview guides that can be used for these purposes [14, 15]. We find this information can provide useful detail on process measures such as the characteristics of the relationship and its perceived impact on the mentor and mentee.

Outcome measures at the individual level (for mentors and mentees) include assessment of academic productivity, such as number of publications and peer-reviewed grants, as well as teaching effectiveness scores or awards. These data can be captured through review of annual activity reports or review of CVs. Similarly, you could collect information on time to promotion and retention of faculty at five and ten years after the mentorship program was initiated.

Overall, we found few tools or strategies for measuring impact of mentorship or a mentorship program. Most studies focused on capturing satisfaction with mentoring or on grant and publication success. These measures may not be optimal for all career paths. For example, for clinician teachers/educators, you could consider assessing teaching awards or teaching effectiveness scores as well as retention and promotion. Similarly, for clinician-administrators you might want to capture leadership positions at the local, regional, national, and international levels.

Designing the methods for evaluating the impact of your mentorship program

Once you've identified the outcome measures, you need to consider your study design or evaluation framework. We encourage use of quantitative and qualitative methods. Quantitative methods can include a randomized trial, an interrupted time series, a controlled before-and-after study, or a cross-sectional study amongst others. It might be difficult to randomize sites or participants to receive mentorship or not but elements of the mentorship program could be assessed in a randomized trial. For example, if you are initiating a mentorship program, you could conduct a randomized trial of participation in a mentorship workshop and determine its impact on productivity and retention of mentors and mentees, or their experiences with mentorship. An interrupted time series is an ideal design to use to assess impact of a mentorship program. In this design, data are collected at multiple points before and after the intervention to determine if the intervention has an effect greater than the underlying trend; the key considerations are to work with an experienced statistician to ensure that sufficient data points are available. A controlled before-and-after study could also be considered. Using this method, one cohort receives access to the intervention and another does not. Outcomes data are collected before and after the intervention in both cohorts. If you are interested in testing an intervention in a single context, identifying a control group which is comparable will double the effort in terms of data collection, but provide a much more reliable answer than a simple before-and-after study. Most of the mentorship studies that we identified in our literature search were cross-sectional studies; these studies include surveys conducted at a discrete point in time, for example, assessing how many faculty members have a mentor. These latter studies have also been used to complete nested cohort studies, whereby faculty members with mentors are compared with those without using outcomes such as productivity or time to promotion. We won't include a detailed description of these various evaluation methods in this chapter and instead refer readers to a clinical epidemiology textbook for further information [16].

Selection of your study design requires consideration of what measurement strategies are feasible to use within your setting; for example, can you conduct yearly surveys of faculty members or yearly reviews of their annual activity reports? What resources will be required for your design? Is this data collection strategy sustainable over the next three years, or five years? Feasibility of the study design also requires that you ensure that data collection is not too onerous for the participants; for example, you may want to consider conducting faculty surveys every two years and supplementing this information with reviews of annual activity reports. Individual interviews can be resource intensive and you may not want to conduct these yearly. However, they can provide a rich source of information over time on experience with mentorship.*

Qualitative methods can complement the quantitative evaluation and provide rich information on the fidelity of the mentorship program (for example, what elements of the multicomponent mentorship education intervention did faculty members actually receive?), and on the experiences of mentors and mentees. Interviews, focus groups, and document analysis (such as reviewing departmental policies) are potential sources of qualitative data. This information can also inform the sustainability of the mentorship initiative and may identify new challenges to mentorship that may need to be addressed by the program; we will discuss this further in the next chapter on 'Scaling up and sustaining a mentorship program'. For additional details on qualitative methods, we encourage readers to refer to a textbook on qualitative research methods [17].

---

* Note that this is a great opportunity for trainees and junior faculty to get involved with education scholarship; for example, departments could invite budding clinician educators to tackle the evaluation of the mentorship program and its subsequent redesign as a scholarly project.

Bottom line and scenario resolution

Evaluating the impact of a mentorship program can target the individual (including the mentor and mentee) and the institution. You should consider quantitative and qualitative methods when developing your evaluation strategy. You also need to balance your interest in evaluating impact with the resources that you have available to collect data over time. Moreover, faculty are bombarded with requests to complete surveys and interviews and you should make sure that data collection is not too onerous for them.

Returning to our scenario from the beginning of this chapter, when you started your mentorship program you developed a stakeholder advisory group with representation from faculty members from different career paths and ranks to ensure that their needs would be met and that the sustainability of the strategy would be considered. You created an evaluation strategy that would include data collection at the individual and departmental level as outlined below.

At the individual (both mentors and mentees) level:

• Survey department members every two years including questions on whether they have a mentor (and their experience with that mentor; Box 7.1), self-efficacy, job satisfaction, job-related well-being
• Review CV/annual activity report for department members every year and extract the following data: publications, promotion, grants, honours, leadership positions. You decide to use an interrupted time series design and use yearly data from five years before the intervention and five years after the intervention.
• Interview department members using purposive sampling of faculty across career paths and ranks. You propose to conduct this in alternate years to complement the survey data and you will explore perceptions and experiences with mentorship (Box 7.2).

At the departmental level:

• Review departmental annual report to determine the number of mentorship workshops held annually and faculty attendance at each of these events.
• Review department annual report to identify the number of divisions within your department that have a mentorship facilitator.
• Review departmental annual report at five and ten years to determine the number of faculty retained at five and ten years after the mentorship program was initiated.
• Review annual activity reports from faculty members to determine the number of new and junior faculty who have a mentor.

You completed the analysis of the data available from the first two years of the program (including the results of the survey and interviews) and presented these data to your department.

Reviewing departmental annual reviews, you report that all of the divisions except for one have a mentorship facilitator. Your team had already flagged this as an issue to explore and found that the mentorship facilitator is on sabbatical and no replacement was named. You were able to remedy this with a quick discussion with the relevant division head.

The survey found that 95% of the new and junior faculty in the department have a mentor, compared with 20% prior to the implementation of the program. Approximately half of the mid-career and more senior faculty don't have a mentor and state they would like one; this interest in mentorship from more senior faculty is increased compared with the results from your survey of faculty before the mentorship program was implemented. Almost half of the department members have participated in at least one mentorship workshop. The majority of department members who have a mentor state that this relationship has had a positive impact on their career and job satisfaction.

The qualitative data reveal that mentors and mentees perceive the relationship to be meaningful and productive. Challenges to the relationship include lack of time for meetings between the mentor and mentee. Some of the participants stated that they were unclear if mentorship was being rewarded in promotion criteria and you highlighted this as an issue for discussion at the departmental retreat.

Overall, you tell your department chair that preliminary data suggests that more department members have a mentor and believe that it has had a positive impact on their productivity and satisfaction. You suggest that more information will be available in three years when you're able to look at impact on productivity, promotion, and retention of faculty using an interrupted time series design. You have also flagged some issues for improvement of the program such as identification of new mentorship facilitators and ensuring that mentorship is incorporated in promotion and tenure review.

Box 7.1 Survey for faculty members

1 Consider whether you believe your mentor has played a role in your career development and success over the last 1 year. Please indicate your level of agreement with the following statements.

	Strongly disagree	Disagree	Neither agree nor disagree	Agree	Strongly agree
a) My mentor had a negative impact on my career development					
b) My mentor had a negative impact on my career success					

	Strongly disagree	Disagree	Neither agree nor disagree	Agree	Strongly agree
c) My mentor had a positive impact on my career success					
d) My mentor had a positive impact on my career development					
e) My mentor and I meet regularly to discuss my progress					
f) My mentor helped me to be strategic about research opportunities					
g) My mentor helped me to be strategic about grant opportunities					
h) My mentor helped me to be strategic about presenting my research at academic meetings					

2 Please indicate your assessment of your current mentoring relationship

i) My relationship with my mentor was excellent					
j) I had adequate meeting time with my mentor					
k) I would have preferred to meet more frequently with my mentor					
l) I would have preferred to meet less frequently with my mentor					
m) I felt comfortable talking about scholarly activities with my mentor					
n) I felt comfortable talking about personal issues with my mentor					

Box 7.2 Sample questions for interviews of mentors and mentees

Mentee interview

1 What is your experience of mentorship that you have received?
2 When and how was your mentor–mentee relationship established and why? (Was it a formal requirement, was it something that you identified as a need and set about arranging, did it "just happen"?).
3 How easy/hard was it to find a mentor and establish that relationship?
4 Were there any barriers for facilitators to identifying a mentor?
5 Do you perceive any barriers when receiving mentorship, e.g. financial, cultural, etc.?
6 In your opinion what can the funding agencies do to overcome these barriers and encourage the success of mentoring relationships? Do you have any advice for them about mentorship?
7 Should the funding agencies create any mentor intervention for coaching mentors or mentees that would help the process
8 Do you believe that mentors should have a formal training or continuing medical education (CME), at least, before they mentor? (If they say information session should be made available should this be made available for Mentee, mentor or both.)
9 Who is your mentor? Name _____ Phone # _____
10 How often do you meet with your mentor?
11 What do you receive from the mentor? What do you discuss with your mentor? What are your expectations of your mentor?
12 What do you perceive as the elements of a successful mentoring relationship? Of a failed mentoring relationship?
13 If you have experienced a failed mentoring relationship what was the impact on yourself and your mentor?
14 Do you mentor anyone?
15 In your opinion what role should the mentor play when mentoring?
16 Can you identify any relevant materials from their organization on formal mentorship programs?
17 What was your mentor's role in preparing your application for funding? What was your experience of mentorship in this process?
18 Do you have any advice for the funder, the university, or others about mentorship?
19 Do you have any other comments to add about your experiences with mentorship?

Mentor interview

1 What is your experience of mentorship that you have received?
2 When was your mentor–mentee relationship established and why? (Was it a formal requirement, was it something that mentee identified as a need and set about arranging, did it 'just happen'?).

3 To what extent is the nature of mentoring relationship formally acknowledged?
4 Do you have any advice for funding agencies about mentorship
5 How would you characterize your relationship with your mentee?
6 What do you perceive as the elements of a successful mentoring relationship? Of a failed mentoring relationship?
7 If you have experienced a failed mentoring relationship what was the impact on yourself and your mentee?
8 Do they perceive any barriers when providing mentorship, e.g. financial, cultural, etc.
9 In your opinion what can the funding agencies do to overcome these barriers and encourage the success of mentoring relationships? Do you have any advice for them about mentorship?
10 Do you believe that mentors should have formal training or CME before they mentor?
11 Have you had mentorship for different aspects of your career, i.e. clinical, research, political, etc.? What are the values of different types of mentors?
12 In your role as mentor, what do you aim to do?
13 In your opinion what role should the mentor play when mentoring?

References

1. Sambunjak D, Straus SE, Marusic A. Mentoring in academic medicine: a systematic review. JAMA 2006; 296; 1103–15.
2. Straus SE, Straus C, Tzanetos K. Career choice in academic medicine: a systematic review. J Gen Int Med 2006; 21: 1222–9.
3. Sambunjak D, Straus SE, Marusic A. A systematic review of qualitative research of the meaning and characteristics of mentoring in academic medicine. J Gen Int Med 2010; 25: 72–8.
4. Curtis P, Dickinson P, Steiner J, Lanphear B, Vu K. Building capacity for research in family medicine: is the blueprint faulty? Fam Med. 2003; 35: 124–30.
5. Wise MR, Shapiro H, Bodley J, et al. Factors affecting academic promotion in obstetrics and gynaecology in Canada. J Obstet Gynaecol Can. 2004; 26: 127–36.
6. Dutta R, Hawkes SL, Kuipers E, et al. One year outcomes of a mentoring scheme for female academics: a pilot study at the Institute of Psychiatry, King's College London. BMC Med Educ 2011; 11: 13.
7. Dilmore TC Rubio DM, Cohen E, et al. Psychometric properties of the mentor role instrument when used in an academic medicine setting. Clin Transl Sci 2010; 3: 104–8.
8. Feldman MD, Huang L, Guglielmo BJ, et al. Training the next generation of research mentors. Clin Trans Sci 2009; 2: 216–21.
9. Abedin Z, Biskup E, Silet K, et al. Deriving competencies for mentors of clinical and translational scholars. Clin Transl Sci 2012; 5: 273–80.

10. Graham ID, Logan J, Harrison MB, *et al.* Lost in knowledge translation: time for a map? J Cont Edud Health Prof 2006; 26: 13–24.
11. Straus SE, Graham I, Wong A, *et al.* Development of a mentorship strategy: A knowledge translation case study. J Cont Educ Health Prof 2008, 28: 117–22.
12. Gusic ME, Zenni EA, Ludwig S, First LS. Strategies to design an effective mentorship program. J Ped 2009; 11: 173–4.
13. Donabedian A. The quality of care. How can it be assessed? JAMA 1988; 260: 1743–8.
14. Straus SE, Chatur F, Taylor M. Issues in the mentor-mentee relationship in academic medicine: qualitative study. Acad Med. 2009; 84: 135–9.
15. Straus SE, Johnson MO, Marquez C, Feldman M. Characteristics of successful and failed mentoring relationships: qualitative study across two institutions. Acad Med 2013; 88: 82–9.
16. Haynes RB, Sackett DL, Guyatt GH, Tugwell P. *Clinical Epidemiology: How to do clinical practice research.* Philadelphia: Lippincott, Williams and Wilkins, 2005.
17. Creswell J. *Qualitative Inquiry and Research Design.* Thousand Oaks, CA: Sage Publications, 1997.
18. Warr PB, Cook J, Wall T. Scales for the measurement of some work attitudes and aspects of psychological well-being. J Occup Psychol 1979, 52: 129–48.
19. Warr PB: The measurement of well-being and other aspects of mental health. J Occup Psychol 1990, 63: 193–210.

Chapter 8 **How can you scale up and sustain a mentorship program?**

Scenario

Following the presentation on the evaluation of the mentorship program that you gave at your departmental retreat, your department chair called you and said she'd like you to address some of the challenges identified in the preliminary data that you presented. Namely, she wants you not only to scale up the mentorship program to offer mentorship to mid-career and more senior faculty members but also to outline your plan for sustaining the program over the next five years. Your mentorship program team is happy to hear this vote of confidence in the program and decides to hold a half-day meeting to brainstorm a strategy.

How do you scale up a mentorship program at your institution?

The extent of the scale-up must be considered. For example, are you planning on scaling up to all the members of your department? Of your entire faculty? Of your whole university? A program that works in one setting or department may not be easily implemented in another. For example, a mentorship program developed for a department with a high ratio of potential mentors to mentees will need to be modified for another department with fewer faculty and lots of potential mentees.

Scaling up the mentorship program may be also necessary if you initially launched it in just one division or institution. Similarly, your initial launch may have targeted one group of faculty members (such as new recruits or junior faculty) with the intention to include faculty in other ranks and career paths if it was successful. Other programs have begun with clinician-scientists and then rolled out to clinician-educators and administrators.

Mentorship in Academic Medicine, First Edition. Sharon E. Straus and David L. Sackett.
© 2014 John Wiley & Sons, Ltd. Published 2014 by John Wiley & Sons, Ltd.

Regardless of the target for growth of your mentorship program, when developing your scaling-up strategy you have to consider the same issues that we outlined when developing your program (as discussed in Chapter 6), namely:

- the needs of the faculty/division/department
- barriers and facilitators to uptake of mentorship and the mentorship program
- how the mentorship program needs to be adapted to these barrier and facilitators.

Moreover, you need to consider the resources required to scale-up the program across the additional divisions or academic ranks. As before, the keys to success include engaging both the relevant targets of your expansion and the people who control the resources necessary for its implementation.

How do you sustain a mentorship program at your institution?

Before a mentorship program is launched, you need to consider sustainability: "The degree to which an innovation continues to be used after initial efforts to secure adoption is completed" [1]. There is no point in developing an elaborately complex mentorship program if there will be insufficient resources (either financial or human) to sustain it. Ominously, Burnham and colleagues reported that just 44% of mentorship programs in the academic health science centres they studied had a budget of $25,000/year and most have less![2]

We did not find any studies that specifically addressed the sustainability of a mentorship program. Sustaining begins with ongoing monitoring of the impact of an intervention, followed by modifying its components and support if its desired impact is reduced over time. We find it useful to consider the ongoing monitoring of a mentoring program as analogous to post-marketing surveillance of drug use: Are new adverse effects of the intervention noted? Are the benefits of the intervention diminishing over time? If so, why is this happening? Answering these questions requires both quantitative and qualitative data. The quantitative data tells you if you're continuing to see the impact you want to see, and the qualitative data identify the factors that might be influencing this impact. For example, perhaps a change in departmental leadership reduced the attitudinal and financial support that was present when you started the program, and led to its decline. Your qualitative data can identify and explain this decline and reveal how you have to address and modify either the attitudes and support at the top or cut back and consolidate the most vital elements of your mentorship program at the "coal face."

Sustainability models typically consider three core elements of process, staff and organization [18]. The *process domain* includes:
- the benefits of the program (from mentorship itself and from participating in the mentorship program)
- the credibility of the evidence (such as we presented in the previous chapter) that these benefits are occurring
- the adaptability of the program over time in response to changing needs of mentors, mentees, and departments
- the adequacy of the monitoring methods and their execution.

The *staff domain* includes training and involvement (are mentors and mentees participating in available workshops?), behaviors (of both mentors and mentees), and support from senior leadership. Finally, the *organization domain* determines whether the organization's goals and culture facilitate mentorship, and whether there is sufficient infrastructure support of mentors and mentees.

The program implementation literature [18] suggests that these factors be consolidated into seven questions that can serve a sustainability strategy:

1   Has the need for mentorship been clearly identified?
2   Do the benefits of the mentorship program outweigh its harms?
3   Is appropriate leadership in place to sustain the mentorship program?
4   What resources are needed for sustaining the mentorship program (e.g. financial, human, infrastructure)?
5   Does the mentorship program align with departmental or institutional culture?
6   What concurrent interventions will be competing for resources?
7   Who are the opinion leaders or champions that can be accessed and mobilized to help sustain the mentorship program?

Bottom line and scenario resolution

Your departmental survey (described in Chapter 7) identified that the mentorship program has stimulated interest amongst more senior faculty in getting mentored. Your team decides to focus efforts on this group and proposes to:
- ask each division head in your department to link faculty with the mentorship facilitator if they don't have a mentor; the annual review with each division member will be the trigger for this
- work with the division head and department chair to ensure that the mentorship facilitator has sufficient protected time to meet this need
- create a workshop for more senior faculty on mentorship challenges
- include mid-career and senior faculty in the qualitative interviews and surveys that are held every two years as part of the evaluation strategy for the mentorship program to determine if their needs are being met.

Your working group has also developed an approach to optimizing sustainability of the mentorship program including:

- Ongoing monitoring of the impact of the mentorship program using the strategy outlined in Chapter 7: you propose to use the data from this process to continually refine the program and to make annual reports to the department chair.
- Ensuring divisional mentorship champions are retained through ongoing financial and other support from the department chair: given that the responsibilities of these individuals have increased because of the scale-up of the program, you ask for additional funding from the department chair.
- Rewarding mentorship in promotion and tenure decisions: your team develops the template (Table 8.1) that will be included in the academic CV and annual reports required by departmental members. You work with the department chair to arrange a meeting with the dean to develop a plan to include mentoring in the faculty's promotion criteria.

Table 8.1 Impact of mentorship activities

Name of mentee	Position of mentee; location	Date	Outcome of mentorship*

*Outcomes of mentorship can include educational courses developed and implemented, grants received, manuscripts published, awards received amongst, others and we suggest you review Chapter 7 for other examples of potential outcomes. Note, that we have deliberately kept this table simple so that data collection is not too onerous for the mentors.

- Developing annual departmental awards for mentors of junior faculty and more senior faculty.
- Developing terms of reference for the mentorship program development group: you offer to chair this program for the next five years, ensuring that new members are brought into the working group for three-year terms (renewable once).

References

1. Burnham EL, Schiro S, Fleming M. Mentoring K scholars: strategies to support research mentors. Clin Transl Sci 2011; 4: 199–203.
2. Davis B, Edwards N. Sustaining knowledge translation interventions, In: SE Straus, J Tetroe, I Graham (eds). *Knowledge Translation in Health Care*. Wiley Blackwell, 2009.

Index

Mentorship in Academic Medicine, First Edition. Sharon E. Straus and David L. Sackett.
© 2014 John Wiley & Sons, Ltd. Published 2014 by John Wiley & Sons, Ltd.

Printed and bound by CPI Group (UK) Ltd, Croydon, CR0 4YY